The Silver/Gray Beauty Book

The Silver/Gray

Photography by George Monserrat

Illustration by Joan Farber-Vernon

Beauty Book

TONY RAY, Beauty Director of La Costa Spa

and

ANGELA HYNES

RAWSON ASSOCIATES: New York

Library of Congress Cataloging-in-Publication Data

Ray, Tony.
   The silver/gray beauty book.

   1. Beauty, Personal.   2. Gray hair.   3. Middle aged women—Health and
hygiene.   4. Cosmetics.   5. Color in clothing.   I. Hynes, Angela.   II. Title.
RA778.R33   1986   646.7'042   85-43089
ISBN 0-89256-306-0

Published simultaneously in Canada by Collier Macmillan Canada, Inc.
Packaged by Rapid Transcript, a division of March Tenth, Inc.
Composition by Folio Graphics Company, Inc.
Printed and bound by Fairfield Graphics, Fairfield, Pennsylvania
Designed by Jacques Chazaud
First Edition

Contents

Acknowledgments

The authors would like to thank the following for their expertise and professional help in preparing this book: Tina Avina, Linda M. Bryson, Collagen Corporation, Mollee Geraty, Dr. Peter Goldman, Judy Hicks, Kevin Nelsen, Jackie Nguyen, Sandi Parmelee, Querida Pearce, Pepi, Katherine Vaz, Warren-Mikal Wrian, the staff at La Costa, and all our makeover models, but especially Maggi Gladden, for the generous use of her home.

Time cannot wither her, nor custom stale her infinite variety.

—WILLIAM SHAKESPEARE

Introduction

We could not have written this beauty book before now. There was no need or desire for it. But it became obvious to both of us, at almost the same moment, that this book was an idea whose time had come. In Tony's case, more and more clients at his La Costa beauty salon started showing up with silver hair who wanted to keep it that way.

"These are bright, beautiful, busy women with families, jobs, and active social lives," according to Tony. "Some of them also are involved in sports—running, golf, tennis, aerobics, weight training. Most of my clients are absolutely stunning women who want to stay elegant and appealing forever. But they don't have the time to laboriously color their hair and maintain their 'roots' every few weeks. And frankly, they don't care to. I think that women who wear their silver hair proudly are doing more than making a fashion statement. They are proving that they are secure in who they are.

"But there's more involved than just letting the gray grow in, and these women had questions. Many, many questions about looking after their hair, styling it, and wearing the right makeup to complement it. I realized that, although there are hundreds of beauty books on the market, these women were special, and there was no guide that met their needs."

Angela's experience was personal. "My hair turned silver when I was twenty-five. At that time I was unique. People would stop me on the street and congratulate me on my 'courage' for not coloring my hair. They always seemed surprised that hair could be both silver and worn fashionably styled rather than in a 'matronly' way.

"A few years ago I began to realize I wasn't being stopped as often. Now I'm just one of many. I see women all the time who have silver hair worn long or in contemporary bobs, even 'buzz' cuts—and they look great. We often nod and smile at each other, acknowledging our membership in an exclusive but growing sorority."

Since we live in a society where the majority holds sway, our perceptions of beauty are changing. Evidence is all around us. Every night on television we see over-forty beauties such as Joan Collins, Linda Evans, Linda Gray, and Stephanie Powers, who, in the teenage-dominated sixties, would have been relegated to playing somebody's mom, clad in an apron and wielding a wooden spoon. Now they portray women who run corporations and steal their daughters' boyfriends!

Glance through the ads in any glossy women's magazine: "Forty is fabulous," says Germaine Monteil, and Tish Hooker, the company's beautiful, silver-haired model and spokesperson, pictured here, proves it. "Sixty isn't what it used to be," states the Ultima II ad, showing three stunning generations of the Alexis family. And the editorial headlines on the opposite pages confirm the fact that yes, Virginia, it is true: You're not getting older; you're getting better.

For all kinds of complex reasons, America is now catching up with what has always been known to be true in Europe—maturity equals allure. Older women today *are* more beautiful than they were in the past.

Fewer women than ever before are confined to the home: almost 60 percent of you go out to work. Your friends and colleagues of all ages provide examples of how to look attractive, as well as inspiration to do so. Furthermore, to some extent, working women are evaluated in terms of the way they look, and that provides additional motivation for maintaining a good appearance. Today's woman is out in the world enjoying a rewarding life in the boardroom—and in the bedroom.

There recently has been a spectacular rise in the older-woman/younger-man phenomenon. Not only are mature women maintaining their attractiveness; they are doing it so successfully that their younger sisters are losing men to them. Joan Collins, Mary Tyler Moore, and Raquel Welch, all are married to younger men. And why shouldn't men find these women a catch? Some dictionary definitions of mature include ripe, seasoned, experienced, expert, adult, and complete: an appealing package indeed!

Women today are positively reveling in the advantages maturity brings. And one of the ways they are doing that is by allowing their hair to go glamorously silver. In fact, several of our makeover models were in their thirties—young for silver hair—but none would dream of coloring what she sees as a definite beauty bonus.

We are lucky enough to be living in an era when beauty is less rigidly defined than ever before. You now tend to choose the hemline, hair length, and color palette that suit you best, rather than living by the unrealistic standards dictated by fashion editors or industry mavens. And many are choosing silver-gray hair.

Some of our makeover models explain why. "My career only took off after my hair turned silver," says June. She feels that her hair gave her an air of sophistication that instilled confidence in the viewers of the television talk show she hosts.

Tish Hooker, Germaine Monteil spokesperson and model

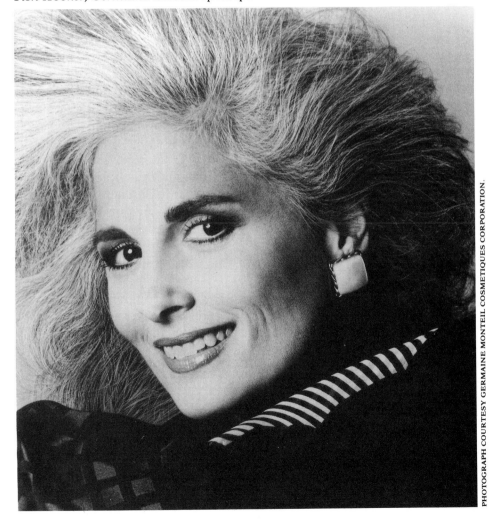

PHOTOGRAPH COURTESY GERMAINE MONTEIL COSMETIQUES CORPORATION.

Judy feels "the silver is me. What would I change it to? Besides, my family likes it the way it is. They encourage me to leave it silver."

"Some women spend hundreds of dollars to have this look. I used to frost my hair to get this effect," says Janet. "It's much prettier now that it's natural."

Today, beauty takes many forms. As cases in point, the women in the pages of this book are all beautiful in different ways—except that they all have silver-gray hair. The other quality we helped them to share with you is the self-confidence that comes from knowing they look *their* very best.

Like you, when they chose to go to silver, they all realized that they needed some new guidelines for glamour. That's where this book comes in. Anything we did to our models, you can do at home—we'll show you how. We are going to talk about the most up-to-date techniques and products available for dealing with the silver-gray stage of beauty.

We will cover the changes in *texture* of your skin and hair; why your favorite colors may no longer look right and which ones will; how to overcome the need to apply a different kind of makeup; what to do about age giveaways such as hands, feet, and teeth.

The news is good. By taking full advantage of all the beauty-enhancing techniques available today—within a loose frame fashioned by genetics and biology—you can be anything you want to be at any age.

Beauty in our society is a woman with an enthusiastic and open-minded outlook who radiates health, vitality, and confidence. All of these are far from being exclusive attributes of youth, but are qualities that can last *forever*, depending on the attitude *you* decide to adopt. Celebrating your silver hair can be the beginning of a celebration of a more sophisticated rest of your life.

Tony Ray
Angela Hynes

PART I

HAIR

1. Heading into Maturity

Hair—it's your crowning glory when it looks great; you want to pull it out by the roots when it doesn't. And talk about temperamental! Hair has the devilish habit of waiting for a special occasion to let us down; yet it can make us feel radiant when we stride out of the hairdresser's with a smashing new "do." We spend hours of our life trying to get our hair to look right, and then, just when we think we're getting a handle on it, our hair starts changing color, texture, and density.

I see an increasing number of women at our La Costa Salon who need to know how to deal with hair that's turning silver, and everything that entails. I always admonish them to throw out their old strategies and to learn *new* ones. But before I give you my "mane event" tips, take a moment to review some brief but all-important hair facts:

• Even as it becomes more delicate with age, your hair is extraordinarily resilient. Yet, unlike your skin, which grows new cells every few weeks, once your hair has emerged from your scalp, it has no facility for renewing itself. It's essentially dead protein!

Hair consists of three parts: the medulla, or minute center of the shaft; the cortex—the thickest part—which holds the pigments; and the cuticle, a protective layer of overlapping cells or platelets (think of fish scales).

• You have about a hundred thousand strands of hair on your head, and their average rate of growth is one-quarter of an inch per month. By the time the ends of your hair reach your shoulders, they are about four years old! During that time, the hair has been subjected to the rigors of the elements, pollution, chemical processing, everyday washing—plus heat drying, brushing, and combing. Imagine what a piece of fabric would look like after that kind of abuse.

Of course, you can cut off any damage or grow it out. And, provided you are generally healthy, your regrowth will be good as new. The condition of your hair is *extremely* susceptible to what is going on in the rest of your body. Thyroid imbalances can wreak incredible havoc: An underactive thyroid can result in brittle, frizzy hair, while an overactive thyroid turns hair lank and greasy. Nutritional deficiencies, such as inadequate iron or vitamins, too, are likely to make themselves apparent via your hair. Any unexplained and sustained change in the condition of your hair might suggest that a visit to your doctor for a checkup is overdue.

But let's say your physical condition is good and you treat your hair with care. You *still* have to deal with the effects of natural aging. Like your skin, your hair is subject to some biological degeneration over the years. But don't despair—this change in your hair *can be a real boon.* Nondescript hair suddenly looks much more striking when streaked with silver; lank, greasy hair dries out; coarse hair becomes more finely textured. And if you don't like the changes, you can achieve anything you want—well, almost anything—with today's marvelous cosmetic technology.

You *can* head into maturity with glorious, shiny, healthy hair. That calls for being aware of *exactly* what's happening to your tresses so you can treat them accordingly.

LEAVE IT TO THE PROS

I've repeatedly stressed the importance of consulting a professional hairdresser, but there's a little of the closet hairdresser lurking in all of us. The temptation to take matters literally into our own hands can be irresistible. But curb your urge when it comes to cutting, permanently coloring, or perming your hair.

Be aware that over-the-counter hair products—particularly colorants—are totally different from formulations that the professionals use. It makes perfect sense, when you think about it, because the pros rely on *much* more sophisticated and potent chemicals.

When you color your own hair, it's a case of a little knowledge being more dangerous than none. Just because you have seen your hairdresser using a tint labeled "Number 5" does *not* mean that you can march into a drugstore, buy the same manufacturer's Number 5 home colorant, and expect the identical glorious results. You'll save a bundle, but trust me when I tell you that this is not a place to pinch pennies—especially since, these days, the best effects are achieved by such subtle procedures as selective weaving and varying shades of highlights. *Not* a chore for the heavy and unskilled hand!

The same applies to perming. It could be that all you need is a body wave or a spot perm. You simply do not have the knowledge and expertise to do the best job, and chances are, your hair will end up fried.

In most of the fifty states, hairdressers have to undergo extensive schooling—usually for about a year—take a state-controlled exam, and obtain a license before being able to practice. But, sad to say, schooling alone does not guarantee quality. We've all had at least one experience in which a rogue hairdresser has infuriated us by charging an obscene amount of money to make us look like freaks. A reputable hairdresser is worth his or her weight in styling mousse!

Here are my tips for finding the perfect hairdresser:

• Ask for referrals. When you see someone with beautiful hair or a knockout style, ask where she had it done. Even if you talk with a stranger on the street, chances are she'll be flattered enough to point you toward her hairdresser.

• When considering a salon for the first time, by all means subject it to an "atmospheric check." If everyone is leaving with neo-punk buzz cuts, or if the place is too intimidating and you don't feel comfortable—head for the door and forget about making an appointment.

• Don't be shy to ask for a price list and for the salon's policy on tipping. Make sure all costs are within your price range. Many salons have special discounts for senior citizens—*ask*, and take advantage of them if you qualify.

• Listen to advice and suggestions from the stylist, but don't be bullied into something you don't want (especially if you're set on staying silver and he's adamant about coloring)! Use the time-honored method of bringing in a photograph of the look you want.

WHEN YOUR HAIR GOES GRAY

Everyone's hair turns silver sooner or later, but the change doesn't necessarily denote advanced age. Many people spot their first silver stragglers in their twenties, others not until their sixties. Two of our makeover subjects—Carey and Charlene—are cousins, who both turned silver in their early thirties. Blame your genes for your exact "silver commencement" age and the eventual percentage of silver you'll have.

Graying occurs when the body slows down—and eventually stops—the production of color pigmentation in the hair roots. Nobody knows why that happens, and as of right now, there is no way to stop your hair from turning silver once your inherited time clock starts ticking. (I'm sure you've already noticed that it happens to your pubic and body hair as well as the hair on your head, but at a much slower rate.)

"Gray" is, in fact, a misnomer, because hair devoid of pigment is actually white. It gives the *illusion* of gray when mixed in with your original color. White interspersed with brown or black hair looks steel or iron gray (unless it grows in streaks,when it contrasts sharply and looks silver). Red, unfortunately, grays the least attractively, and can appear gingery. Blond looks less golden and becomes more platinum—the most subtle change.

Apart from genetics, there are one or two other reasons (uncommon, I might add) why hair turns gray. For instance, there are a few—*very* few—instances of hair turning white overnight as a result of emotional trauma or physical shock.

Some scientists think that a deficiency of vitamin D and some B vitamins may contribute to graying. This is consistent with the long-held belief of health-food aficionados that consuming vast quantities of black-strap molasses will retard, or even reverse, graying, because the substance is rich in those nutrients. I certainly don't recommend such a method of hair coloring, because molasses is also brutally rich in calories! It isn't worth turning into a beach ball, even on the off-chance that you'll stay brunette slightly longer.

The biggest question facing the woman who starts to notice appreciable amounts of gray is whether to color—or not to color. When you have up to about 25 percent silver in your hair—the "salt-and-pepper" effect—it's decision time. There are numerous temporary and permanent colors available: Companies such as L'Oréal and Clairol specialize in tints and rinses for convering gray at home. You should be able to match yours with no trouble . . . but you should cover your silver with a coloring a couple of shades *lighter* than your hair, to blend it in subtly. Remember that you will have to touch up the regrowth every few weeks—silver roots give a far more aging appearance than a headful of silver hair.

One alternative: Have your hair highlighted with additional streaks to *play up* your emerging silver. Or lighten your base color a shade, to make the silver less obvious: auburn to strawberry blond, medium ash brown to light ash brown, and so forth. Just remember—the key to coloring once your hair begins to go silver is always to think *lighter*, not darker.

I know some lucky women whose silver grows in beautiful streaks over their ears or in the middle of the forehead. Why would anyone want to cover this enormously attractive feature? I can't imagine anything more striking—other women pay good money for exactly that effect! Think about it; it's long been considered striking and distinguished on men. Why not on women?

Once your hair is more than one-quarter silver, I recommend that you not try to mask it. Your skin tone usually gets paler as your hair lightens. Your original hair color may now look too dark or have a hard, "dyed" effect. Think how beautiful actress Elizabeth Taylor looks in her fifties, now that she has allowed her raven hair to lighten around her face. Start reveling in your silver, and be proud of what it declares about you as a mature woman. Remember, youth is no longer the only game in town.

At every stage in going silver, your hair will assume a new level of beauty. When it's 50 percent silver, it will give your whole appearance a softer look; at 75 percent, the effect will be light and bright; when it is 100 percent white, it will look silvery and almost ethereal.

I'm assuming, though, that you can keep that pure, white look. Silver hair is susceptible to "yellowing." Here are the basic facts, plus my suggestions for dealing with this problem:

• It should come as no surprise that the sun can burn your hair: The havoc that Old Sol wreaks on your skin has received much publicity recently. Any sustained period of suntime can give your white hair a flat, yellow cast. Furthermore, the sun's blazing heat can cause permanent damage to your hair by drying it out and making it brittle.

Protect your hair under a wide-brimmed hat. Consider slicking your hair back in a "wet-look" style with a rich conditioner when you are on the beach or by the pool . . . this offers protection *and* conditioning at the same time. Many hair-care products now have a sun screen incorporated into their formulas (look for PABA on the list of ingredients).

• This may surprise you: Some shampoos, conditioners, and styling aids such as spray, mousse, and gel can cause yellowing. "Build-up" has become a hair-care industry buzz word describing this condition. Resi-

(continued on page 15)

CARE AND MAINTENANCE

Day-to-day hair care *should* be a simple matter of cleaning and conditioning, but the one-two process is definitely complicated by the plethora of different products on the market. Let's have a look.

The Right Way to Shampoo Your Hair. Hair cleansing used to mean getting rid of the dust, dirt, and oil on your scalp, but

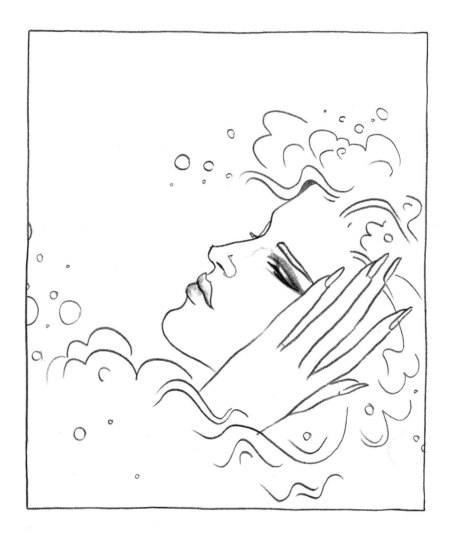

these days, it can also mean washing out pollution, conditioners, mousses, gels, and sprays.

Washing your hair in the shower every day is an acceptable regimen *if* your hair is oily. Oily hair can become lank and rank if not washed regularly. But as years tick by and your hair becomes drier—or if your hair has always been on the dry side—every other day is quite sufficient. Don't stick to old habits if your needs have changed.

I'm always bewildered by the assortment of shampoos available. Manufacturers have left no stone unturned in developing a formula for every conceivable eventuality: processed hair, colored hair, frequently washed hair, heat-dried hair—you name it.

If you've already discovered a product that helps your condition, great. Go ahead and use it. Bear in mind, however, that your hair is dead tissue and cannot absorb or assimilate most of the exotic ingredients many formulas promote. At best, additives such as protein and balsam coat your hair shafts to give them a little bulk, but only until the next time you shampoo.

Look for a simple shampoo with a short list of ingredients. Then dilute it by pouring half the shampoo into an empty bottle and topping up both bottles with water. Nearly every shampoo on the market is far harsher than a woman with delicate or dry hair needs, and leaves a buildup of film residue. Diluted shampoo cleans just as effectively, while cutting down on these negative effects. It is also easier on your wallet!

Whether you wash your hair every day or every other day, here is the La Costa Shampoo Strategy:

• Gently brush your hair to untangle it and loosen dust and deposits of spray or setting aids.

• Wet your hair in warm water. Let the water pour over your head for a couple of minutes before shampooing. This makes it easier to wash out setting aids.

• Pour a measure of diluted shampoo about the size of a quarter into your hand. Rub it between your palms and apply to your hair. Vigorously massage your scalp with your fingertips—not your nails!—being sure not to miss your hairline. Swirl the suds through your hair with care. Remember that your *scalp* needs cleansing more than your hair.

• Rinse your head thoroughly to get all the shampoo out, but don't take too seriously the old adage "rinse till it squeaks." Chances are, you have stripped too much natural oil from your hair if it's giving you that kind of back talk. (The feel of your hair, soft and uncoated but not like guitar strings, tells you when it is free from soap.)

The hard water common in many parts of the country might make it difficult to wash soap residue completely from your hair. Try rinsing with a mixture of three parts water to one part vinegar, or two cups of water with the juice of one lemon.

• Apply instant conditioner if necessary (see the next section). Massage through your hair, not on your scalp, and leave on for a minute. Rinse as with shampoo.

• Pat excess water from your hair with a thick towel. Rubbing will tangle your hair and make it difficult to comb out.

Conditioning Your Hair. Conditioner should help untangle matted, wet hair, control static, and smooth down the cuticle of your hair shaft in order to promote shine and softness. Contrary to popular belief, conditioner cannot repair damaged hair—but it *can* make it a little easier to handle.

As with shampoo, there is a wealth of brands for every possible hair type. But conditioners usually fall into one of two categories: *instant*—also known as cream rinses—and *deep*.

Instant conditioners are applied after shampooing, left on the hair for about a minute, and then rinsed out. I *do not* recommend them for everyone. If your hair is fine, they'll make it limp and hard to style. And if you have oily hair, they'll just make your condition worse.

Instant conditioners are a boon for taming hair that is dry, wiry and thick. (If your scalp is oily but your hair is lifeless at the ends, apply the cream rinse to the parts that need it.)

Deep conditioners are rich in oil. Usually you apply them to wet hair and leave them on under a shower cap or warm towel for about fifteen to thirty minutes—*terrific* for dry, brittle, overprocessed hair. Most manufacturers recommend that you use them only occasionally—once or twice a month. Sound advice! Don't fall into the "more is better" trap, or you'll have an oil buildup that will make your hair dull and heavy.

When it comes to conditioning, let your hair be your guide. Is it silky and bouncy? Your conditioning program is right. Is it sticky and dull? Try going without a conditioner for a couple of washes and see how your hair feels, or switch to another product.

due from one or a combination of these products can collect on your hair and dull or discolor it.

To counteract buildup, give your hair a break whenever possible. On weekends or on vacation, just wash your hair with a mild shampoo, such as Neutrogena, and let it dry naturally. You might also try switching shampoo brands from time to time, because one brand's buildup can be washed out by another shampoo. Also, your hairdresser has professional formulations to take care of the problem—ask about them the next time you go there for a haircut.

• Need another reason for giving up smoking? The same nicotine that discolors your fingers can turn your hair yellow in the front, especially if you are a heavy smoker. What can I say? Stop smoking!

• The gas burner on a stove is another offender. On occasions when you "slave over a hot stove" for a long period of time, wind a pretty bandana around your head to protect your hair.

• Atmospheric pollution can also distort your hair color. This is a tricky situation to avoid—you don't want to stay indoors for the rest of your life! If you live in a place where the pollution problem is particularly severe, be scrupulous about washing your hair frequently, so that chemicals don't accumulate.

If your yellow tinge persists despite your precautions, combat the condition with wash-in rinses—Clairol's Silk and Silver line is excellent. These days, you can also get styling mousses that—on a shampoo-to-shampoo basis—can tone down your color while giving your hair body and fullness. Roux's Fanci-Full Color Styling Mousse comes in two colors—White Minx and Silver Lining—that will do the trick.

It's shades of ash, white, platinum, and silver, possibly with faint blue or lavendar undertones, that will counteract the yellow. But beware of the "blue-rinsed" old lady look! If you're contemplating a permanent tint, I strongly advise you to have your color corrected professionally—or you could end up singing the blues.

CHANGES IN HAIR TEXTURE

As well as turning silver, your hair will become drier as you age, for much the same reasons that your skin dries. Hormonal changes, particularly a decline in estrogen after menopause, slow down the production of sebum (the natural, lubricating oil that smooths down the cuticle of each hair shaft) in your scalp. This isn't bad news if your hair has been oily and limp since adolescence—your condition has finally normalized. But if you've suffered from brittle, breakable hair all along, your hair now will

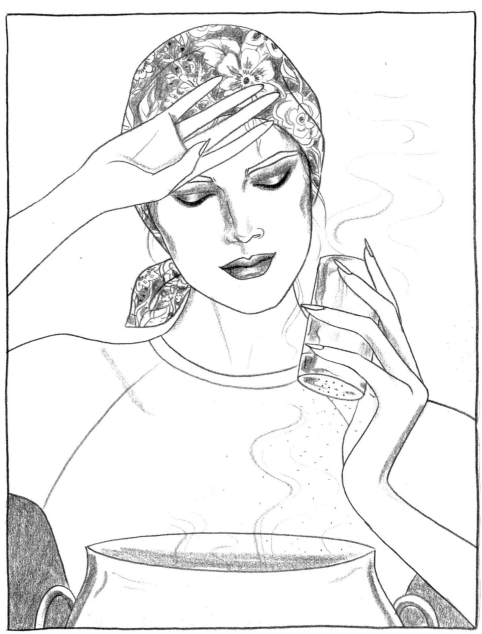

Protect your hair from "yellowing" when cooking over gas.

be quite fragile. Since it's the oil content of your hair that makes it lustrous, drying causes it to lose some of its natural sheen.

With each successive decade, your individual hair shafts also lose some thickness. They are most bulky when you are in your twenties, but by the time you are about seventy, your hair is approximately 20 percent thinner—you're back to "baby" fine once again!

I stress *compassion* in handling your hair now. A little care and kindness can make all the difference between dull, thin hair and healthy-looking, voluminous hair.

• Forget that old wives' tale about brushing your hair a hundred strokes every day. That may have been a valid concept in days when women washed their hair infrequently and needed to distribute through-out the hair the oil that was building on the scalp—oil that in turn protected the hair from the rigors of the brush. But if you jump into a hot shower at least once a day, as so many of us tend to do, you strip your hair of its natural oil with shampoo and heat. All that brushing is no longer warranted.

When you use a brush to style, opt for a soft, natural-bristle type. It costs a little more, but the results are worth it. Do *not* brush your hair when it is wet. Instead, untangle it with a wide-toothed comb. Buy one with rounded ends, so you won't break your hair.

• Heat is more drying to hair than anything else—and we all inflict it on our hair with great frequency. I'll cover styling methods in detail in the next chapter, but it is important to say here that hair dryers—both hand-held and hood types—should be kept on a low heat; hot curlers and curling irons should not be left in your hair for more than the minimum time they need to be effective; and you should give your hair a break from these devices as often as possible. Go ahead and let it dry naturally!

• Extremes in the weather and overheated or air-conditioned indoor environments can sap precious moisture from your hair. Many of the common-sense precautions you take to protect your skin will also benefit your hair.

• Chemical processing, such as bleaching, dying, perming, and straightening, drastically alter the structure of your hair. Although most modern formulas have built-in conditioners, these processes invariably leave your hair dry and fragile. *Never* expect your hair to withstand more than one chemical onslaught at a time. Have either a perm or a color, but not both.

I can't help but emphasize—again!—that these potentially damaging processes should only be carried out by an experienced professional hairdresser.

• Exercise generally benefits your hair enormously, by stimulating the flow of nourishing blood to the scalp. But if you work out regularly, you probably perspire more than your sedentary friends. Rinse out this salty sweat as soon after exercising as possible.

Although swimming and other water sports are excellent exercise, pool water is not your hair's best friend. The chlorine in pools is a bleach, and that means drier hair or distorted color. A bathing cap is mandatory wear for the regular swimmer, but since water still leaks in, you should take other precautions as well: Wash your hair and rinse it thoroughly after every dip. There are some shampoos that contain special dechlorinating agents. Ultraswim is an excellent choice. Find it in your drugstore or beauty-supply store.

WHEN YOUR HAIR BECOMES THINNER

Male hair loss receives so much press that we forget how anxious and unhappy *women* can become at the thought of hair loss. Luckily, more often than not, these fears are unfounded: We all lose about ten to thirty hairs a day, which regrow, under normal circumstances. One of the few trials nature doesn't inflict on women is baldness! At least not the kind of male-pattern baldness that afflicts so many men. Some women, however, are genetically programmed to experience slight thinning after menopause in the same places as men—the temples and crown.

A more common cause of hair loss in women is the habitual wearing of styles, such as a ponytail or a chignon, that literally pull the hair out by the roots. Frequent use of heavy curlers, pin-on hair pieces, or hair ornaments might also cause trouble. Simply discontinuing the damaging habit will stem the loss of hair, and in a relatively short time your lost locks will grow back.

Or are you one of those people with the nervous habit of inadvertently yanking on your hair, twisting or pulling at it when you are upset or anxious? Well, stop it! This condition actually has a scientific name—trichotilomania—and I've seen women in my salon who have irregular patches of hair loss as a result of this habit.

Hair loss also can be related to trauma, either physical or mental. An event such as an automobile accident or the death of a loved one can cause hair to fall out about three months after the occurrence. The hair will grow back in time, as your system recovers from the shock.

Some medications, too, can cause your hair to thin. If you are experiencing hair loss that you cannot account for and are taking some kind of medicine, ask your doctor if there is a connection. Ill health, bad nutrition, and fad diets are other culprits that can trigger hair loss.

Creative hair styling springs to the rescue when it comes to thinning hair. Don't make that awful mistake—many men are guilty here—of growing it long and trying to cover the thin spots. It looks awful—but no one has the heart to tell the wearer. Short, well-cut hair stands out from the head and looks fuller. A very light body perm, professionally applied, will help to fluff up your hair, as will the use of styling aids such as mousses and gels.

If your hair loss is severe, consider wearing a wig. Human-hair wigs obviously look most like the real thing, but they're also the most expensive. Enormous strides have been made recently in the manufacture of synthetic wigs—they're lightweight and natural-looking. Some even come with open-weave caps through which you can pull hanks of your own hair to blend with the synthetic fibers.

Having a wig custom-made is expensive, and I don't believe it's usually necessary. Just take your "off the peg" model to your stylist and have it professionally fitted, cut, and styled to suit your face.

The base of your wig will absorb oil from your scalp, and the hair becomes soiled from atmospheric pollution just as natural hair does. Don't, therefore, neglect to keep your wig fresh and odor-free. Wash it frequently according to the manufacturer's instructions, or ask your hair stylist for wig-care tips when he or she is styling it for you.

2. Style and Error

We all believe that our hair's texture and condition imposes styling limitations: oily and lank? Forget about long hair. Thin? Don't even *think* about a perm. Fine? Cut it blunt, not layered—and so on. Add to this the notion that we must compensate for structural flaws in our faces with the right hairstyle. Then there are all those rules. You know the ones I mean: Older women shouldn't wear their hair long. . . . Softness around your face will hide wrinkles. . . . Upswept hair gives your face a lift. On top of that, you have to take into account individual hair quirks such as curliness or cowlicks, plus your life-style, manner of dress, and personal preferences, not to mention the prevailing fashion.

It's no wonder so many women come into my salon with absolutely no idea of what would be becoming to them. You'd need a computer, a slide rule, and all the hair stylists on Fifth Avenue to obey all these dictates. I'm going to give you some sound guidelines in a moment, but before I do, the first and most important law is: Don't ever be afraid to break the rules! That's because a style can be technically all wrong, but if it "fits" you and makes you feel good, it's perfect.

These days, there's much more freedom to break the rules, thanks to the sophisticated styling aids on the market. Conditioners, mousses, gels, sculpting sprays, and "air" perms—not to mention styling brushes, curling irons, and about seventeen different types of rollers—all allow you to achieve almost any style you want, regardless of your hair's condition.

I encourage women who've found their dream hairstyle *not* to be afraid to stick with it—with perhaps a gentle "updating" nod in the direction of fashion. Actress Shirley MacLaine is a perfect example: Ever since she started making movies in the 1950s, she has had a short, gaminlike haircut. She's kept her trademark look but always stayed in style *by varying the details*. Some years it's almost boyish; other years it's longer and wispy on the nape of her neck.

Whether you take this approach or go in for drastic changes every season, you might still be confused about which hairstyle will make you happiest. The hundreds of hours I've spent in my salon getting women to that launching point has produced a number of guidelines.

SELECTING YOUR HAIR LENGTH

Hair length is far more than a matter of inches—it's an emotional subject! The way you perceive yourself—frankly feminine, sensual, businesslike, dull, lacking in confidence—is often revealed by your hair. We have so much ego invested in our hair that a drastic change in length can be quite shocking.

• Short is in the eye of the beholder. Take it from someone who's been caught in this dilemma many times: Your idea of a short cut may not be the same as your hairdresser's. Do you mean mid-neck length? A close-cropped, boy's cut? Clip pictures from fashion magazines of what appeals to you, and bring them to your hairdresser. *Don't* just fall back on that old line, "Do whatever you think is best, Pierre." It makes my job so much easier when a woman happily takes responsibility for the way she wants to look!

Extremely short silver hair can look severe, even mannish. Buzzing and spiking, which have been in vogue for most of the eighties, are just too hard for a face that has softened in color and texture. (And if you have put on some weight in the last few years, a cropped cut can make you look like a "pin head.") Fortunately, these styles are now last year's news. What's replacing them? Softer, *classic* looks, full and smooth, with a polished image.

I'm not saying you can't wear your hair very short *if* it looks tailored and sophisticated. Short styles can be high impact and are an excellent means of accentuating good facial features and the shape of your head. But do evaluate yourself honestly!

Probably the most flattering short style for you will have the look and feel of length. That's not as contradictory as it sounds. Just leave the

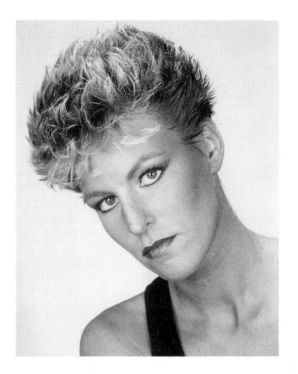

Very short silver hair can look stunning—if you have the features to carry it off.

top longer than the back and sides: As a bonus, feathery bangs will camouflage lines on your forehead (and bangs of all lengths are *in*). Alternatively, keep it short on top but let your hair grow longer on the sides and on the nape of your neck, so that it wisps around your face . . . a *great* ploy for detracting from a less-than-perfect chin line.

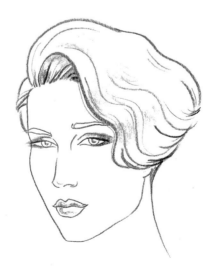

Short cuts that have length and softness on top usually are more flattering than hair cut in a masculine style.

Short can be a no-fuss option for curly hair. Curly hair tends to need less upkeep than straight hair, because it grows out tousled—a style in itself. That's good news for those who neglect to get a trim as often as they should (you know who you are)!

A bob—hair cut one length in a straight line between ear and chin—is a chic look for short hair, and one that is making a big comeback. This polished style is a particularly flattering means of showing off beautiful coloring, such as silver streaks.

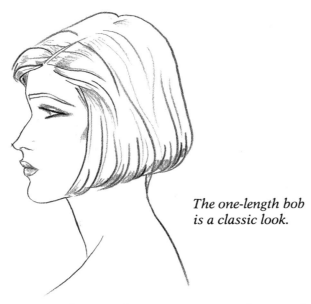

The one-length bob is a classic look.

Short hair is much more low-maintenance than medium or long hair. Just "wash and wear"—step out of the shower and let it dry naturally. Do you have a hectic life-style? Are you a sports aficionado? You'll be happiest with this option.

Let's say you're ready to grow out a short cut. Get through that dreaded in-between stage and compensate for not-quite-right length by keeping your hair in perfect condition—silky and shiny. Curb the temptation to cut off straggly strands that are driving you crazy. Have them trimmed professionally. Even when you are letting your hair grow, you need regular cuts to coax it into your new style.

• I define "medium length" as between chin and shoulder. If I had to generalize, I'd say that medium is often the most flattering length for all women, but especially for those with silver hair . . . and it's certainly the most versatile. I discovered that many of our makeover models had medium-length hair out of choice, and I really did not need to effect any drastic changes in order to give them their best new look.

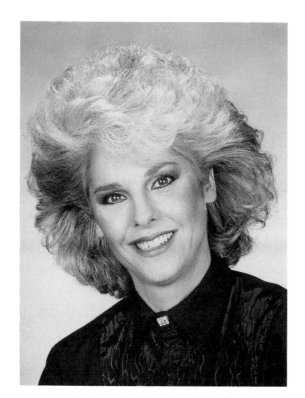

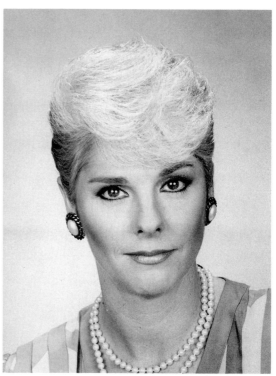

One medium haircut, three different moods.
First a loose, casual look; next a businesslike
French twist; finally a glamorous, upswept style.

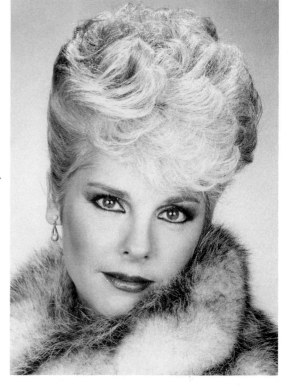

24

But please get a good, stylish cut. The biggest danger with medium-length hair is that you can end up looking matronly instead of sophisticated. Like short hair, medium-length hair needs to be trimmed regularly to avoid becoming straggly. *Beware of small, rigid waves or tight curls—* these are extremely dated looks. Sleek, blunt cuts that graze your shoulder are always elegant, while beveled or layered cuts can be soft and feminine. Medium-length hair offers the option of being worn pinned up, or you can pull it softly back. The short, sleek ponytail at the nape of the neck is very much in vogue.

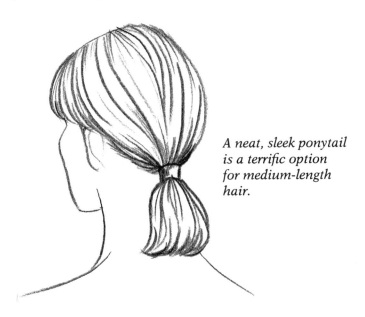

A neat, sleek ponytail is a terrific option for medium-length hair.

• You probably associate long hair with youth. That presents two schools of thought: Since you are mature, you should not wear your hair long, *or* long hair will help you look more youthful. I think that once you have an appreciable percentage of silver, you're better off with a medium style, but not because of the old cliché that it's unseemly for older women to wear their hair flowing below the shoulder. It's because your silver hair is probably dryer and less lustrous than it once was. If your hair is glossy and in great condition, there is no reason why you shouldn't show it off by growing a mane. But you're definitely a rarity. Most long silver hair looks coarse and unruly.

Long styles worn loose fall better if they are layered—the dead weight of one-length hair can pull out style. A little styling gel or mousse at the roots will lift and fluff long hair. Steer clear of styles parted in the middle; they just drag your features down—the last thing you want.

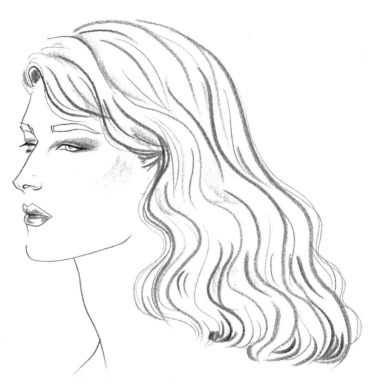

Loose, long hair should always be soft and wavy.
Straight, long hair drags your features downward.

You're better off wearing long hair swept up in a twist or chignon—stunning on mature women! These styles will show off your hair color and give your neck a beautiful line.

Pin up your long hair softly; don't drag it back across your scalp or fashion it into a tight knot—both looks are reminiscent of a matronly schoolmarm. Keep the bulk of the hair on the back of your head. Curls beehived on top don't work!

Hair grows a little more slowly with every passing decade. But don't make the common mistake of cutting your hair less frequently in order to preserve the length. Long hair needs to have the dry—and often split—ends cut off to keep your hair looking healthy.

Many women today lead lives that don't allow time to deal with long hair. It takes longer to wash, condition, dry, and style, and skipping a washing is fatal to your overall grooming. Tying your locks back in a "nonstyle" is not the answer, either. Unless you really have the time to devote to keeping your long hair looking truly sensational, take the plunge and treat yourself to a smashing new easy-care cut.

HOW TO PICK THE RIGHT STYLE
FOR YOUR HAIR TYPE

A fact of life: We always want what we don't have. That's certainly true when it comes to hair. Curly tops long for flowing, silky manes; straight-haired women would die for a mass of waves. I encourage women to enjoy what they have, but if you don't, certain techniques can give you what Mother Nature didn't. You silver-haired women with either straight or curly hair will find you have certain advantages and disadvantages.

• Naturally curly hair might lose some of its spring in time. Be prepared to rethink how you handle your hair when this happens—a style you've worn successfully for years might start to look lackluster. Get your hairdresser to adapt a new style to your new hair texture.

Or try supplementing your own curl with a permanent. Perms use strong chemicals that destroy the cuticle layer of the shaft and penetrate the cortex of your hair, breaking down its very structure. Therefore, proceed with care when your hair is dry, sparse, or colored. It is absolutely taboo even to contemplate a perm within several weeks of having your hair bleached or treated with a permanent color.

Fortunately, perms are light-years ahead of where they used to be. Techniques have become much improved—solutions tend to be gentler, and there are formulas for every type of hair. Many hair salons are offering "air" perms, which eliminate one of the chemical steps, and are thus *much* kinder to your hair.

You don't need to perm your entire head anymore, either. Weave a perm into a particularly flat section, or perm just the roots, the underlayers, or the ends.

Although new options in home perms are available, have your hair permed professionally. First, because your silver hair needs special handling where chemicals are concerned, as a result its texture and coloring (don't forget that chemicals can give your silver hair a yellow cast). Second, because your perm needs to work together with your cut to create the desired look.

Don't want a perm? Blow dry your hair into a straighter style. Curly hair with noticeable amounts of silver appears wiry and coarse even when it's not. Smooth hair reflects light better than curly hair, so if your tresses have become a little dull, a straight style will look shinier, particularly if you have a high percentage of silver or a light original color.

• If you have naturally straight hair, it will now come into its own. Silver hair is often best shown off in sleek, straight styles or deep, soft waves. Take advantage of the growth pattern of the silver to create dramatic effects.

• If your hair is thinning, do not wear straight styles with a part. The scalp that shows will emphasize the problem. A slightly tousled effect, or a short style with a body perm at the roots to lift and fluff your hair, suits you better.

• Straight styles need frequent attention. Dry, flyaway ends are more noticeable when your hair is supposed to be silky. Regular trims and the correct amount of conditioning are a must.

That's my general primer on selecting the right length, but here's a quick rundown on specific ways to pick the look that's just right.

Take your facial features and shape into consideration when picking a hairstyle. Remember that your face changes with time. You might be thinking of yourself as the chubby-cheeked teenager you once were, when in fact the years have revealed terrific bone structure!

Study yourself very carefully in the mirror—full on and in profile—to assess your strong and weak points. Better yet, get a friend to take some Polaroid pictures that you can study objectively. Prominent jaw? Narrow forehead? Great cheekbones? Beautiful eyes? When you go to the hairdresser, you can discuss your strong and weak points with your stylist, so that the two of you can come to a mutually pleasing decision about what looks best.

A *square face* needs soft bangs that are either feathered or cut longer at the sides and shorter in the center. Steer clear of the straight-across variety, which emphasizes the squareness. De-emphasize the severity of your jawline by choosing a soft, wavy, medium-length cut.

A *round face* does well with height on the crown and a bare neck, for an illusion of tallness and length. But if your hair is long, don't drag it back—that accentuates your face's fullness. Wear gently upswept hair, leave some soft tendrils at the nape of your neck. Bangs brushed to the side can also take away some of the roundness.

A *heart-shaped face* needs a medium-length cut. Sweep your hair back behind your ears, where your face is fullest, to show off your cheekbones; then aim for fullness from ears to chin, to add width. Soft bangs are a big plus. Part your hair on the side for a nice shift of balance, and *don't* pull your hair back off your face.

A *diamond-shaped face* has a jawline like that of the heart-shaped face, so follow the same guidelines. But you should also try wide bangs, which will create the appearance of a forehead. Don't bare your forehead and brow area completely—you want to camouflage their smallness or narrowness.

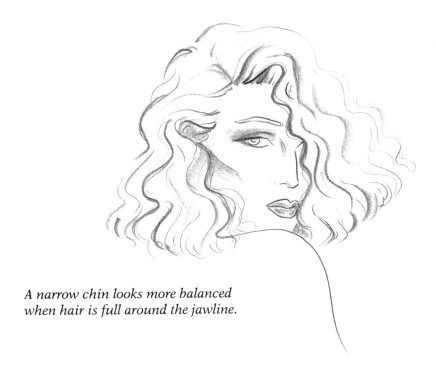

*A narrow chin looks more balanced
when hair is full around the jawline.*

    A long face requires a medium-length, full-on-the-sides cut. Long, straight, hanging hair only makes your face seem drawn. Avoid flatness—go for curls, layering, anything that will break up the long line. Wear a pretty scarf tied bandana-like around your hair, to flatten the crown and give the illusion of width.

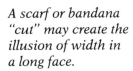

*A scarf or bandana
"cut" may create the
illusion of width in
a long face.*

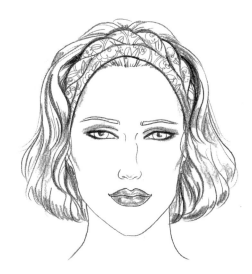

STYLING AIDS CAN SOLVE
MANY HAIR PROBLEMS

New products that proliferate in the beauty industry invariably reflect current trends. For instance, in the 1960s, when long, natural hair was the fashion, most innovations occurred in conditioning preparations. In the 1980s, more elaborate styles, which evolved from spiky punk looks, and a parellel swing toward tailored styles, led to the introduction of sophisticated setting aids that allow you to manipulate your hair with ease.

Have you been wrestling for years with limp, fine hair that never held a set? You'll find these aids a boon. Some of them almost allow your hair to defy gravity! Silver hair that has lost some of its zing can get a real lift from these styling products, and as an added bonus, many of them help control static electricity and contain sunscreens.

A few words of caution. First, most of these products contain large amounts of alcohol, which is very drying to your hair. Unfortunately, it's a necessary ingredient, but check the contents to find brands where alcohol is low on the list, and is therefore in smaller quantities. You'll usually see it written as SD alcohol 40, isopropyl alcohol, or cetyl alcohol.

Second, although these styling aids are formulated to be washed out, daily use can mean the kind of buildup that leads to dullness and distortion of color. Try to take a break from them when you can. Also, switch brands from time to time.

Mousse is one of the most exciting innovations to appear on the hair-care market in recent years. Used in Europe for some time before it came to the United States, mousse is now a staple in all salons and most of our bathrooms, replacing those old-fashioned setting lotions, which leave your hair sticky.

Mousse is a liquid that, when shaken and dispensed from its can, has the appearance and consistency of shaving foam. Squirt a measure about the size of a small egg into the palm of your hand and smooth it onto your hair. The foam disappears as you comb it through. Use mousse on either wet or dry hair and style with a blow dryer, or set with rollers. Any way you wield it, mousse adds volume and fullness that lends itself to soft, natural-looking styles.

There is one exciting innovation in mousses. Both Vidal Sassoon's Colorific and Fanci-Full's Color Styling Mousse let you completely change the color of your hair *for just one day.* So if you get tired of your gray but don't want to make the commitment to change permanently—or even semipermanently—these products can make you a redhead, blonde,

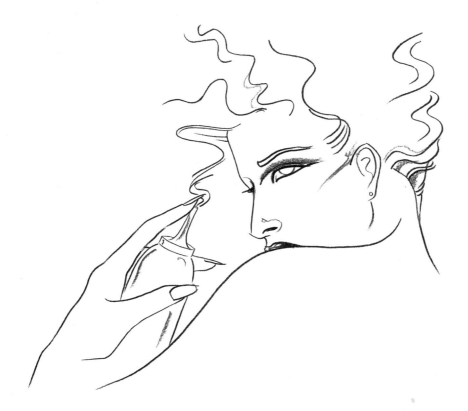

or brunette while they hold your style. And they shampoo right out the next time you wash your hair. You can also use them to add just a "flash" or streak of color when dressing for a special occasion.

Sculpting lotions, glazes, and gels are variations on a theme. They come in different consistencies, from bottled liquids to thick gels in a tube. Apply them to either wet or dry hair, and reactivate between shampoos by spritzing with water.

When used on wet hair prior to styling, sculpting lotion gives a firm set, with defined waves and curls. Apply it to dry hair to achieve a shiny, "wet" look. Gel is ideal for giving flat hair a lift: use your fingertips to apply just to your roots. Sculpting lotions and gels also enable you to separate your hair into wisps and delicate points.

The major disadvantage of gels for silver-haired women? They'll darken your hair, and they're a little too heavy for thin, fine hair, and weigh it down.

Hair spray, like perms, has also come a long way in recent years. The newest are billed as *sculpting sprays*. Paul Mitchell, Vidal Sassoon, and Sebastian all make them. You'll wonder how you got along without them!

They're extrafast-drying, hold until you brush them out, wash out much more easily than old lacquers, and come in pump rather than aerosol dispensers—better for the ecology as well as your health.

Beware of using spray to produce hard, "done" sets that have no natural movement. Such styles are aging and matronly. Use hair spray in moderation on contemporary styles: a spritz to slick hair back behind your ears, a spray to help fluff up your bangs, a squirt to hold a chignon in place—that's all you need!

TAKE ADVANTAGE OF APPLIANCES

Good-bye and good riddance to the days—or rather, nights—of sleeping face down in the pillow because your hair was full of spiky curlers. Annoying on your neck—and not so hot for romance, either. Thank heaven for those appliances that guarantee an elaborate style in minutes while you're rushing madly about in the morning. But if you have dry or fine hair, you must use them with discretion, because overuse can result in even drier, damaged hair.

A critical point: Your hair is somewhat protected from heat when it is wet, and most likely to be damaged by heat when it is dry. So monitor your hair while you are setting it, and stop using the appliance while your hair is still slightly damp. As often as possible, take a break from heat-generating appliances and let your hair dry naturally.

When using a hood or salon-type dryer, gradually reduce the heat as your hair dries. Start out on the highest setting; then turn it down a few notches after about five minutes. Continue this process until it is on the lowest setting for the last five minutes or so. Better yet, emerge from under the dryer while your hair is still slightly damp, carefully take out the curlers, and let it finish drying naturally before you comb it out.

Blow dryers are probably a busy woman's best friend, but her hair's worst enemy. If used *incorrectly*, they strip your hair of its natural moisture, leaving it prone to breaking. Delicate silver hair is especially vulnerable.

When drying hair in sections, hold the dryer at least six inches away from your hair, and do not direct the dryer onto a section for more than a few seconds at a time. Allow a section to cool off before you go back to it.

Never use the hottest setting on your blow dryer. Hand-held dryers often come with nozzle attachments that concentrate the hot air for faster drying. Throw that away at once! Get a diffuser attachment if you wear your hair in a curly or tousled style.

Definitely turn down the heat when you use styling mousse or gel.

DON'T BLOW IT!

Used with caution, your blow dryer can be a remarkably versatile tool for styling your hair. Today's fashion extremes of sleek, smooth hair or casual, tousled styles are easily achieved with this indispensable tool. The stylists at La Costa suggest the following to achieve up-to-date looks:

• For full, casual hair, bend over from the waist and blow your hair dry upside-down. Use your fingers to "rake" your hair forward—the *opposite* direction from its natural growth. When it's almost dry, squirt on a little hair spray just at the roots, stand up, and flip your hair back. Carefully arrange into the desired style.

• To use the "scrunching" technique for a shaggy, sexy look, apply styling mousse to damp hair, then loosely grab handfuls of it. Play the dryer on them on a low heat. When your hair is dry, smear a little more mousse between the palms and run lightly over the surface of your hair to separate strands gently for a soft, tousled effect.

• Add volume by attaching a diffuser to your dryer, and partially dry your hair while pushing it around with your fingers. Then take off the diffuser and dress the hair as usual with the dryer and a round styling brush.

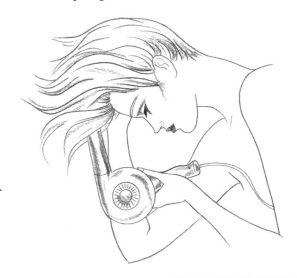

Blowing your hair upside-down can create great volume.

Intense heat literally "bakes" such products onto your hair shaft, making them difficult to wash out. Your hair ends up like straw!

As with hood dryers, don't blow your hair until it's bone dry. This is especially true if you are planning a double whammy, by styling your hair with hot rollers or a curling iron afterward. I recommend avoiding that kind of one-two punch entirely. Towel dry your hair instead, let it finish drying naturally, and then use your hot rollers. If time doesn't allow such a leisurely pace, towel dry your hair, and then whisk your dryer around your hair at its lowest setting to half finish the job. Complete the drying process naturally, until your hair is only slightly damp, and then use the rollers.

• Don't use hot rollers every day. They are brutal on the ends of your hair, which are the dryest parts to start with. Save rollers for occasions when you need a special curly "do," or on days when you are really pressed for time.

Hot rollers should never be left in your hair for more than ten minutes: That is *plenty* of time to do the job. Use the kind that you can fill with water or a conditioning liquid and will set your hair with steam. They are infinitely kinder to your hair. Also, choose special spray-on setting lotions formulated for use with hot rollers. Clairol's Kindness is good.

Put your rollers in and take them out with care; most are heavy and have a tendency to tug at your hair. If your hair constantly gets snarled on hot curlers, wrap perm papers, strips of tissue, or even squares of toilet paper around the ends of your hair before you roll them. After you have removed the rollers, let your hair cool before brushing or combing it.

• Curling irons are both better and worse for your hair than hot rollers. Better because you cannot keep them in your hair for nearly so long—who wants to hold a curling iron in place for ten minutes? Worse because they reach a much higher temperature to compensate for the brief time they have to effect the curl.

Curling irons are very handy for occasional use to give your bangs a flip or add a little lift to the hair on your crown. Wrap your hair smoothly around the barrel, curl it down, taking great care not to touch your scalp, and hold for a count of twelve. Unwrap carefully, and leave your hair curled until it cools down.

When shopping for a curling iron, buy one that has multiple heat settings, and always use the lowest. As with hot rollers, some brands use steam, and these are definitely worth the little extra they cost. Most irons come in sets, with screw-on barrels of different sizes. Find one that has a nonstick coating, just as you get on cookware.

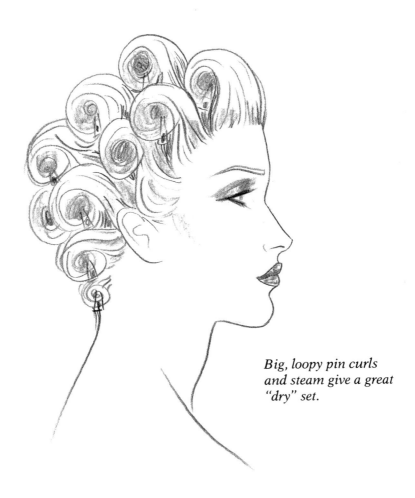

*Big, loopy pin curls
and steam give a great
"dry" set.*

• If your style needs daily curling, invest in a set of old-fashioned sponge rollers from a variety store. On the in-between mornings when you don't wash your hair, roll it dry in the curlers. Alternatively, set your hair in big pincurls, not flat against your head but standing upright, almost as if your hair were wrapped around invisible rollers.

Keep your hair away from the stream of water in the shower by directing the nozzle downward, or take a quick, warm bath. The steamy air in the bathroom will set your hair. By the time you are dressed and made up, your hair will have cooled and dried. If, however, your hair is hard to curl, and steam alone doesn't do the job, comb a dab of mousse through your dry hair before you set it. You're ready to face the world with an all-day style!

TOPPING IT ALL OFF

Be *very* careful about ornamentation for your silver hair. Anything too bright can overwhelm your color—and anything too fussy can look inappropriately girlish.

• Restrict ribbons to dark-colored, Chanel-type grosgrain bows, and *only* to tie long or medium-length hair at the nape of your neck. Forget about pastel, chiffon, or lace ribbons and Alice in Wonderland-style headbands.

• Flowers are similarly iffy. A single gardenia tucked into a

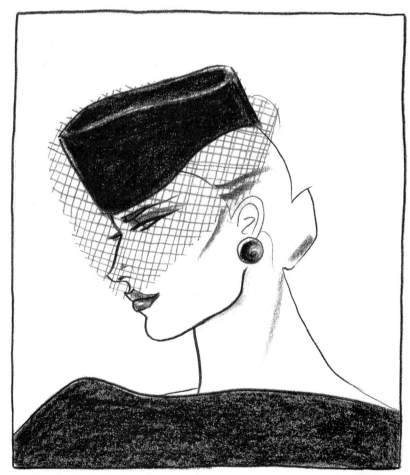

Cocktail hats are big fashion news. Wear one with panache.

chignon might be dramatic, but steer clear of spring-like or bridal-type flowers.

• Scarves can be drab and matronly if tied under your chin à la Queen Elizabeth of England. And save the kerchief tied at the back of your neck for when you tackle housework. Instead, casually twist a pretty scarf and tie it bandana-style at your hairline. If it overwhelms your face or appears as a dark halo, jettison the idea. The effect should be a soft accent at the front of your hair.

• Combs—tortoiseshell, ivory, jeweled—are among the most timeless and classy ornaments you can wear in your hair. Use them to hold up your French twist or to sweep your hair back off your face to show off your cheekbones.

• A mature woman really comes into her own under a hat. A hat can be wonderfully sophisticated, and you can wear it with a panache that no teenager could ever have. Small hats act as an accent and an accessory; big hats are a true statement. The general rule is: The bigger the hat, the more it should blend in with the rest of your outfit.

Extravagant cocktail hats are currently very much in vogue. Little pillboxes tilted rakishly . . . veils over the eyes . . . black berets with a jeweled brooch pinned on the side . . . brocade toques . . . all are being seen out on the town.

PART II

SKIN

3. Facing Facts About Skin

magine the pleasure of having luminous, fresh-looking skin for a lifetime. It *can* be yours no matter what your skin's condition now. Every day women walk into the beauty salon at La Costa with less-than-perfect skin—career women who claim they are too busy to pamper their skin, women who think their silver-gray hair has given them a license to "let themselves go," sportswomen who are resigned to the inevitability of a leathery hide.

Untrue!

After placing themselves in our experts' hands, by the end of their stay at the spa, these women can see a noticeable improvement.

We don't keep our secrets to ourselves! Our clients leave armed with knowledge that will enable them to continue the improvement at home—and we are going to share this with you.

Flawless skin is one of your most crucial beauty assets. And of the twenty square feet of skin that swathe your body, the few precious inches that cover your face are the most important in terms of how you are seen by others—and by yourself. Your face is your presentation to the world.

When it comes to divulging age, your face can be a cruel deceiver. Mistreat it, and your facial skin can look physically years older than you are chronologically.

The most important area of your skin in terms of appearance is the one that time hits hardest. Compare the skin on your face to the skin on your buttocks—undoubtedly, the skin on your derriere will be smoother and clearer. It will show none of the stereotypical signs of aging. Yet both sets of skin are the same age.

The reason for the difference is simple. Much of the degeneration that occurs on your face over the years is *erroneously* blamed on time. On the contrary, it's years of abuse—often in the name of beauty—and adverse environmental conditions that cause our *exposed* skin to age. The real culprits are sun, wind, excessive heat and cold, stress, smoking, alcohol, poor nutrition, facial habits, yo-yo weight loss, pollution, detergents, and some cosmetics. Take heart! They all are elements over which we can exercise some control—if we know how. And this book will tell you how.

Starting here, you are going to take a fresh look at skin care, focus on your individual needs, and zero in on result-producing beauty regimens.

There are two kinds of aging: biological and environmental.

BIOLOGICAL AGING

Biological—or natural—aging has no real set pattern: When it occurs depends on your genetic makeup. Just as hair begins to turn silver anywhere from twenty to seventy in different families, so does skin begin to show lines at different ages. A look at your grandparents, parents, and older siblings, will give you an idea of what you can predict.

Regardless of your personal time clock, there are four inevitable major changes that happen to your face with time. Let's consider what they are and how to deal with them.

How to Fight Wrinkles

To understand wrinkling and what you can do about it, here's a quick, refresher biology lesson on skin. Don't skip it! The more informed you are, the better equipped you'll be to deal effectively with the problem.

The dermis is the deep underlayer of living tissue that houses the blood vessels, sweat and oil glands, hair follicles, and nerve endings of your skin. It is built from a network of proteinous fibers called collagen, which is what makes young skin smooth and plump. These fibers are bound together by another protein called elastin, which is what gives skin its resiliency. Over time, collagen fibers thin out, and elastin begins to stiffen and lose its elasticity. Consequently, the dermis shrinks and the epidermis—or outer layer of skin—now too big for it, collapses into cracks and creases. *Voilà!*—a wrinkle is born.

This process accounts for cosmetic companies' inclusion of collagen and elastin in their skin-cream formulas in the past few years. These creams do a wonderful job of improving the surface of your skin—which is, after all, the part you *see*—by smoothing the texture and making it light-reflective. But they cannot actually *reverse* wrinkling.

Peter M. Goldman, M.D., Assistant Clinical Professor of Dermatology at UCLA School of Medicine and a private practitioner, whose client list includes some of the most beautiful faces in Hollywood, points out that nature has designed skin to be a barrier. Therefore, cosmetic additives don't reach the dermis, where wrinkles originate. Because you can't reverse them, prevention of wrinkles is essential. How can you prevent them?

Dermatologists stress that the dermis must be nourished from the bloodstream. A healthful diet rich in all the necessary vitamins and minerals, plenty of water, and exercise to increase your circulation will give your skin its best fighting chance of warding off lines.

Hedge your bets! Feed your skin from within, and soothe it on the outside with products rich in collagen. At La Costa, we recommend a thirty-day program undertaken two or three times a year, in which you gently pat liquid-soluble collagen onto your face and neck after cleansing at night and in the morning. Our collagen (you can order it through the mail; for a catalog, write: La Costa, 2100 Costa Del Mar Road, Carlsbad, CA 92008) comes in ampoules and is made exclusively for us by Arvel. La Prairie's Cellular Cycle Ampoules and Germaine Monteil's Life Extrême Nutri-Collagen Concentre are similar, excellent products.

These treatments are pricey—no doubt about it. But you only need use them a couple of times a year, ideally when the seasons change. Amortized over the year, the cost per day is small, for remarkably big results.

When Skin Changes Texture

Does your skin seem to be getting drier as you get older? If you answer, "yes," you are in the majority. How parched your skin gets depends largely on the skin type you were born with. Skin that is oilier than normal also tends to be thicker and can stay beautifully smooth well into your fifties. Lucky you! You're getting your pay-off now for all that acne you probably had to put up with as a teenager.

Delicate, dry skin that looks so translucent when you are in your twenties can age much faster than oily skin, and may even start to develop a network of fine lines in your early thirties. It is imperative that you nurture this kind of skin throughout your lifetime.

Why does your skin get drier? There are two main reasons:

• Slowed-down cell renewal. With each passing year, your body loses its capacity for continual cell repair and renewal. Consequently, your skin cells are older, thinner, and less moist than they once were. They tend to slough off in irregular patches, and leave you with dry, flaky skin that looks dull.

Once again, the cosmetic industry rides to the rescue. Technicians at the La Costa labs were among the pioneers in cell-renewal technology. Now many of the major beauty houses have night creams (your cells are busiest while you sleep) that help in the regeneration of cells. Estée Lauder's Night Repair Cellular Recovery Complex is one we especially like. Consistent use of such a cream improves the surface appearance of your dry skin.

• Hormonal changes. It's the oil (or sebum) skin exudes that forms a barrier to hold moisture on your skin. Production of sebum is largely controlled by the female hormone estrogen. At menopause, when levels of estrogen decline, your body only produces about 60 percent of the sebum it did before. Without its natural protector, skin therefore becomes more susceptible to the drying effects of the elements.

A great deal of controversy has arisen in recent years about the inclusion of synthetic estrogen in cosmetic formulas. The uncontrolled absorption into the bloodstream of this powerful hormone has been known to cause severe side effects. For that reason the reputable cosmetic houses have dropped it from their formulations.

The controversy about hormone creams has been nothing compared to the furor over estrogen replacement therapy (ERT). Twenty years ago, this was being hailed as a virtual fountain of youth—high doses counteracted many menopausal symptoms, and had a wonderful side effect . . . dewy, fresh skin.

But it quickly became apparent that ERT was linked to certain types of cancer. Today doctors are more cautious about prescribing oral estrogen, give much smaller doses, and only allow its use for a limited period of time. If you are on ERT for medical reasons, you probably will enjoy an improvement in your skin tone. But you would be foolish to undergo this type of therapy simply for the sake of your skin—the down-side risks are too great.

Concentrate instead on using a good moisturizing lotion that will take place of the lost body oil and do the same job the oil does—that of holding moisture on your skin. (More about moisturizers in the next chapter.)

Dealing with Discoloration

Changes in skin color are a normal part of maturation. You might have to deal with some of these:

• "Liver" spots. Of course, these have nothing at all to do with your liver. These small, irregular brown patches are sometimes the result of uneven sun tanning. But they also can be caused by hormonal changes affecting the pigment cells in the skin. They tend to be triggered when your body is undergoing upheavals such as pregnancy or menopause.

"Fade" creams such as Porcelana and Esoterica help even out color by bleaching the skin. But apply them carefully—they also can lighten the area around the spot, causing a "halo" effect. A dermatologist can offer a permanent solution by freezing discolored patches with liquid nitrogen, under local anesthetic. One of the surgical rejuvenation therapies, such as chemical peeling or dermabrasion, also will take care of the problem. If the spots are not too large or dark, you can simply cover them with makeup. (More about all of these techniques in later chapters).

• Hemangiomas. These are common little blemishes that many women get on their faces, necks, or chests in their thirties. Raised red bumps with tiny areolas, they tend to look like permanent pimples. Although they are harmless, it's worth getting rid of them for beauty's sake. A dermatologist can zap them in his office with an electric needle or a laser beam in fifteen seconds—the procedure is virtually painless and totally effective.

• Broken capillaries. The network of fine red lines that can appear on your cheeks is also a candidate for quick and painless removal in the dermatologist's office by the application of an electric current via a very fine needle.

• Dark circles under the eyes. Most of the skin on your face thickens slightly with age. Not so the skin around your eyes—it becomes thinner. This delicate skin lets the blood-rich dermis show through, which is what causes the dark-circle effect. The tendency toward dark circles is a hereditary trait.

You can cover the circles with makeup if you know the correct technique. We will show it to you later in the book. Also, be sure to get plenty of rest, because burning the candle at both ends definitely makes the condition worse.

• Skin pallor. As you mature, you sometimes look paler than you did in your youth. This is because—as when your hair turns silver—your body is not producing quite as much pigmentation, and also because your circulation is not as brisk as it once was. Brighten up a pale face by getting plenty of exercise, and by the clever application of blusher.

In any event, this lightening of your skin usually coincides with the silvering of your hair, so the whole effect is beautifully harmonious.

Facts About Sagging

Over the years, gravity takes its toll on your face. On the positive side, at about the same time, your facial structure often becomes more apparent, and you discover glamorous cheekbones and beautiful eye sockets that you never knew you had!

Many of the remedies that are thought to counteract gravity fall into the category of myths. Facial exercises are a good example. The muscles of the face are attached to the skin, unlike many of the larger muscles in the body, which are attached to bones and joints.

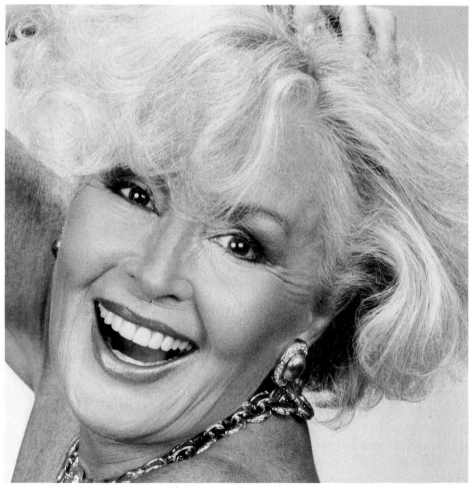

Proof positive that a sparkling smile can be your most flattering accessory

Every time you laugh, cry, eat, or talk, you work them out—they may get the most exercise of any muscles in your body! It is this constant repetitious movement that, in fact, determines where the lines and creases will form on your face. Far from rejuvenating your looks, facial exercises only make the problem worse.

Similarly, facial massages, vibrators, and accupressure treatments do little to retard the sagging of your muscles. But they do no harm, and they help many women feel pampered and relaxed—so why not?

One of the best gravity-beaters is smiling! There is more to it than the mere fact that a happy face has a youthful sparkle. Smiling turns up the corners of your mouth, lifts your cheeks, and crinkles your eyes—all of which counteract the downcast look of sagging muscles.

The only surefire way to reverse gravity is to have a full or partial surgical face lift. We will explore all the options there are in Chapter 9.

ENVIRONMENTAL AGING

Do you like to have a deep suntan? Do you live in a windy city? Do you smoke? Are you always dieting to lost ten pounds? Does your life-style involve a lot of travel? Are you worry-prone? These are just some of the questions to ask yourself if your skin looks older than it should.

Though there is no turning back the clock, the news is good. You can put the brakes on any further deterioration of your skin—at any age. *Right now* you can make some simple changes in your habits to ensure that in another twenty years your skin still will be lying about your age—but this time in your favor! Also, with a little know-how, you can vastly improve the appearance of your skin *regardless* of its condition.

The following pages reveal some of the most common environmental beauty-beaters and tell you what you can do to counteract them.

Beware of Too Much Sun

Coco Chanel has a lot to answer for. It's reputed that she came home from a Mediterranean vacation in the 1920s with a suntan, and started the whole fashion of having bronzed skin. Until then, a tan meant you belonged to the peasant classes and worked out of doors. But overnight sun-browned skin became a symbol of the leisure class, and the melody lingers on: These days, tan is still equated with rich, chic, and sexy.

Because La Costa is a resort as well as a spa, many of our clients are sports fans—they come for tennis, golf, and swimming. So we see first-hand what the sun can do over a period of time if you don't take proper precautions. But we also have become adept at dealing with the problem—and you can, too!

It's ironic. What's regarded as a healthy glow is, in fact, the result of your skin trying to protect itself from sun damage. Tanning is a process of *retaliation*. At its first exposure to those burning rays, the skin begins to produce a brown substance—melanin—that rises to the surface as a self-imposed partial barrier to the damaging effects of the sun. Melanin thickens the surface of the skin and absorbs some of the sun's radiation, so that it cannot penetrate to deeper tissues. That thickened skin can look leathery and tough—but it doesn't have to.

Sunlight *does* have some beneficial effects. It makes you feel healthier (the sun's warmth can relieve aching muscles and joints), younger, more sensual, and more energetic. Scientific studies have shown that sunlight counteracts depression. The sun also triggers production of vitamin D, essential for the absorption of calcium. But you can get all the sunlight you need in order to reap these benefits just by going about your daily business: no need to spread-eagle on the beach at high noon.

On the minus side, the sun is responsible for about 90 percent of all nonnatural aging changes to the skin: wrinkling, weathering, broken blood vessels, and blotchiness. That's not to mention skin cancers such as melanoma, which is most common in women in their forties, and basal- and squamous-cell cancers, which result from thirty to forty years of cumulative sun exposure and occur in older people.

Ideally, we need a new arbiter of fashion such as Coco Chanel to create a craze for porcelain complexions. Tanned skin and silver hair are not particularly compatible, so perhaps some "glamorous gray" will emerge as a trend-setter! But probably it will be a couple of generations before our attitudes toward tanning change. Some public-spirited fashion magazines already have made the decision not to use darkly tanned models in their photo spreads, and the American Cancer Society, with its "Fry now, pay later" advertising campaign, is doing a sterling job in trying to educate us about the dangers of acquiring that burnished look.

In the meantime, you may feel that a light tan makes you look your best. If so, here are five ways you can take the sting out of the sun's rays—and prevent any further premature aging of your skin.

• *Wear a sunscreen every time you go out.* You get more than half of the ultraviolet radiation you absorb just from your normal routine. Don't assume that just because you are not in the habit of lounging by a pool or on the beach in a skimpy bikini, you are not at risk from the sun.

Sunscreens act by either *absorbing* or *reflecting* the sun's harmful rays. PABA (short for para-aminobenzoic acid) is one of the most effective absorbent sunscreens made, and is what you usually find in lotions today.

The best-known of the reflectors is zinc oxide—it works well, but most of us don't want to walk around with an opaque paste on our faces.

Check our chart to find the right sun-protection factor (SPF) for your skin, and wear it under all your makeup, including your moisturizer. A number of companies are making nonoily lotions especially for the face. Coppertone has a whole line called For Faces Only, and Lancôme's Conquête du Soleil Specifics for the face are excellent. Also, look for PABA on the list of ingredients of your moisturizer and foundation. Many manufacturers are now listing it in their cosmetic products.

SUNNING BY THE NUMBERS

The Skin Cancer Foundation has broken down skin types into six categories, depending on how skin reacts in the sun.

1. Very fair, with red or blond hair and freckles: always burns, never tans
2. Fair-skinned: burns easily, tans minimally
3. Fair- to medium-skinned: usually burns first, tans gradually
4. Medium-skinned: minimum burning, always tans
5. Medium- to dark-skinned: seldom burns, always tans
6. Black or very dark-skinned: never burns, tans darkly

Recognize yourself? Now check your number against the sun-protection-factor (SPF) guide below, to see what type of product you should use in the sun.

(NOTE: An SPF tells you how many times longer you may stay in the sun while using protection than if you were *not* using a sunscreen. So if a sunscreen has an SPF of eight, you can stay in the sun eight times longer than you could if you had no protection. The higher the SPF, the greater the protection.)

Skin Type	Degree of Protection Needed	SPF Needed
1	Ultra	15+
2	Maximal	8–15
3	Extra	6–8
4	Moderate	4–6
5 and 6	Minimal	2–4

PABA and PABA esters can cause allergic reactions in some women. If you're one of them, look for alternatives. Biotherm has a line of sun-protection products that is PABA-free, and Clinique makes a good foundation that has a maximum sun block, using opacity instead of chemistry.

Don't forget to apply sunscreen at all times to your neck (it's often neglected), the tip of your nose and the tops of your ears (highly vulnerable), and your lips (they contain no melanin). Protect these sensitive areas with a total sun block of 15 or more SPF. In their Sundown range, Johnson & Johnson have a sunblock stick in SPF 15 that is handy for applying to these regions.

When you get serious about sunning—at the pool or beach, or playing outdoor sports—apply a sunscreen to all exposed parts of your body. Your arms, legs, and back are obvious, but also remember the backs of your hands, tops of your feet, and your decolletage. Make sure it's a waterproof formulation, and religiously follow the directions for reapplying.

Those formulations with a cream or oil base tend to be longer-lasting than those in a water or alcohol base. But oil-based sunscreens have been

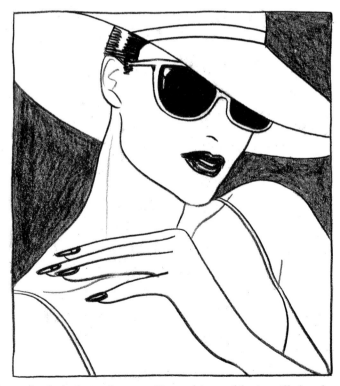

Be a shady lady in the sun. Your skin and hair will thank you.

known to cause irritation, rashes, or excessive perspiration in some women, so experiment and choose one that works for *you*. All the major manufacturers make both oily and nonoily formulations. A rule of thumb is that products called "lotions" are oil-free, while creams are not, but check the labels.

A fairly new development in the sun-care world is the "tan accelerator." This is a lotion that speeds up the production of melanin when you apply it before sunbathing. This means that you spend a shorter time in the sun to get a deeper tan. But it is *not* a sunscreen, and won't protect you from burning. Estee Lauder makes one that you apply for three days before sun exposure, Clinique calls its Suntan Encourager, and Lancôme incorporates an accelerator in some of its Conquête de Soleil line.

• *Cover up.* Wear a wide-brimmed hat or a visor if you are going to be in the sun for any length of time. Always take an umbrella to the beach or choose a spot that has some natural shade. There are hats and visors available today that filter out the burning rays of the sun and let the tanning rays through—they are much in demand at the La Costa boutique.

Most importantly, invest in a good pair of sunglasses, and always wear them outside. What's good? Sunglasses should screen out 75 to 85 percent of ultraviolet rays: If you choose mirrored lenses, you get even more protection. Glass is preferable to plastic, because it screens out more harmful rays.

When it comes to color, dark gray gets the nod, because it filters out both ultraviolet and infrared rays. Brown—the runner-up—lets in the infrared, which can make your eyes red and irritated. Forget about glasses tinted orange, yellow, blue, lavender, or rose—they are only fashion accessories, and offer little protection. Also inadvisable are gradated lenses and those that darken and lighten according to the amount of available light. They don't protect as well as solid-tinted lens.

When buying sunglasses, try them on in front of a mirror. You shouldn't be able to see your eyes if the lens is dark enough to be effective. Wraparound styles or ski-goggle-type glasses are especially good in strong sunshine, because they stop light from coming in at the sides that makes you squint. But don't wear them for driving, because they can impair your peripheral vision.

• *Take atmospheric conditions into account.* Altitude greatly intensifies the burning power of the sun. For every thousand feet of elevation, ultraviolet light is increased by about 4 percent. If you are in a mile-high location, such as Denver or Mexico City, you will burn 20 percent faster than on the beach in Florida. It's essential that you take greater precautions when you are in the mountains.

Similarly, ultraviolet rays increase, the closer you are to the Equator. So if you take a tropical vacation, you need extra protection, even if you are used to the sun.

Water, beach sand, snow, and light-painted surfaces all bounce ultraviolet rays up at you. This reflected radiation can add between 25 and 100 percent to the sun's burning power. These insidious, secondhand rays can burn you even when you are sitting in the shade, and if you are wearing a hat, you will not be protected from the rays that are hitting you from below.

• *Hydrate.* A sunning trick popular in Europe is to spray the body frequently with water—Evian conveniently makes an aerosol can of its mineral water. This is an excellent idea, which helps keep you cool (via evaporation) and replaces some of the moisture that your skin craves. But be sure to reapply your sunscreen if the water eventually washes it away.

It's also important that you have something to drink close at hand to counteract the moisture you loose as you perspire. Water and fruit juice are your best bets, with alcohol and caffeine drinks the worse. They actually are diuretics!

• *Take extra precautions if you get your tan in a tanning salon.* New technology is making these establishments commonplace, and we tend to minimize their dangers. Manufacturers of the latest sun lamps claim to have eliminated from their artificial "suns" most of the ultraviolet-B (UV-B) rays associated with sunburn and cancer, and only hit you with tanning ultraviolet-A (UV-A) rays. Dr. Goldman points out, however, that "anything that tans, injures." He likens tanning in a salon to smoking a filter-tipped cigarette: it's preferable but still not good for you.

Certainly these machines do allow you to skip the sore, red phase and let you go straight to the golden tan stage. Also, some dermatologists recommend them for the relief of certain skin conditions, such as psoriasis. But the American Medical Association has issued a warning against the dangers of the high-intensity UV-A rays used in tanning salons. They penetrate more deeply than UV-B rays and can damage the connective tissues and blood vessels in the dermis layer of the skin, aging it prematurely.

UV-A rays can also trigger toxic reactions in people taking certain medications—including antibiotics—and cause cataracts in those who don't cover their eyes properly. *Always wear the opaque goggles provided.* Furthermore, studies with animals suggest that UV-A rays may act as cancer promoters by inhibiting enzymes that otherwise could repair cells damaged by UV-B rays.

So proceed with caution. At La Costa, we strictly regulate the use of our tanning booths. Keep your artificial sunning to about thirty minutes a week, and use these salons just to maintain a *little* color (that's all you need with silver-gray hair).

If you can't be persuaded that pale is interesting, think about getting your tan from a bottle, by using a cosmetic bronzer that you apply like foundation and clean off at night. There are a number of excellent natural-looking ones on the market: Try Indian Earth or Revlon's Pure Radiance. It's the only really safe way to get that glow.

Less successful are the fake tan compounds (such as QT or Sudden Tan) that contain a chemical called dihydroxyacetone, which reacts with your skin to produce an unnatural color that lasts for several days, and looks particularly unattractive against silver hair. Also pass on tanning tablets. They are illegal in this country, but some people are importing them from Europe or Canada and selling them privately. They can be toxic if taken in high doses, and the orange color they produce is ugly!

How Heat Affects Your Skin

There are, of course, more sources of heat than the sun. Sitting too close to a blazing fire, cooking over a hot stove, ironing, and using a blow dryer can strip moisture from your skin and cause broken capillaries on your cheeks. Apply lashings of moisturizer and use common sense when you are exposed to these insidious heat sources.

How Cold Affects Your Skin

Winter packs a double whammy to your face. Cold air cannot hold humidity, so the frigid outdoors saps moisture from your skin; and artifically heated, stuffy rooms complete the job. This can make anyone's face parched, but for skin already prone to dryness, it can cause severe roughening and possibly itching.

Furthermore, harsh winds, rain, and snow can cause damage in the form of broken blood vessels. Why? The body reacts to chilled air by sending blood to the skin to keep you warm. This influx of blood to the capillaries—the body's smallest transporters of blood—can cause them to break. The result is a network of tiny red lines on your cheeks. These can be treated by a dermatologist, but why get them in the first place?

When the temperature starts to drop, you need to take some face-saving measures. Here are four hot tips for beating the cold.

• *Don't wash your face as often in winter.* Do it once a day instead of twice. Washing strips the skin of its natural, protective oils, which help trap moisture. When you *do* wash, use tepid rather than hot water. Also, avoid soap in winter. Cleanse with a creamy lotion.

• *Use a winter-weight moisturizer.* Apply it twenty minutes before you hit the outdoors. Otherwise, your skin will be "wet" from the water in the moisturizer, and prone to chapping. You need an emollient moisturizer that will create a barrier against evaporation. You might find that you prefer to use a light coating of night cream during the day in winter. (You will, of course, be using it lavishly at night.)

Lips need special protection. When the air is dry, you tend to lick your lips; then the moisture evaporates, drying them even further. It's a vicious cycle, which can leave you with cracked, sore lips in the short term and damaged tissue in the long term. Before you go out, apply one of the widely available lip balms that contain emollients and sunscreens, such as Chapstick or Blistex. Carry one in your purse or pocket and reapply whenever your lips feel the slightest bit dry.

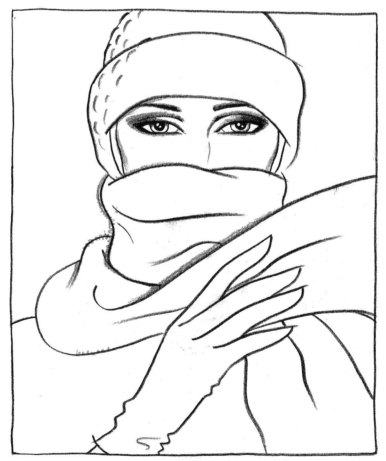

Cover as much exposed skin as you can in harsh winter conditions.

• *Wrap up.* Cover as much of your face as you can in harsh winter conditions. Wear a hat pulled low over your forehead, a muffler wrapped around your lower face, and glasses or goggles on your eyes. Ideal wear would be a ski mask.

• *Moisturize the air!* Increase the humidity in your home and place of work: Artificial heat dehydrates your skin terribly. A relative humidity of about 40 to 50 percent is ideal. How do you achieve that? Start by running the heat down a few degrees—most buildings are overheated in the winter.

To add more moisture to the air you can buy a commercial humidifier. They're available for under twenty dollars in a drugstore or department store. (Pay a little more for a vaporizer and add eucalyptus or menthol oil when you have a cold.) This works well in a small room, but is less effective in a large space—the moisture simply dissipates.

If you don't want the expense of buying one of these devices, the old standby, a saucer of water on the radiator, works just as well. Place a full saucer on each unit or in front of your space heater and top it as the water evaporates.

The most pleasant and healthy method of keeping your air humid? Have a houseful of green plants. If you keep them well watered, they will keep your air well watered also!

PERSONAL HEALTH HABITS AND AGING

Smoking Is Harmful to Beauty and Health

According to the United States Surgeon General, "smoking is the chief single avoidable cause of death in our society and the most important health issue of our time." Apart from that, it gives you wrinkles!

There's a twofold reason for this. One is obvious: Years of pursing your lips to inhale and squinting your eyes against the smoke eventually will etch lines in your face. Secondly, doctors believe that smoking causes a stiffening of blood vessels, strangling vital blood supply to the dermis. As a result, smokers tend to suffer sallow, dry skin, which ages more quickly than that of nonsmokers.

Habitual smoking can discolor the skin of your face and hands, your teeth, and your hair. Silver-gray hair is especially susceptible to yellowing from smoke.

There's one surefire remedy for all these problems. Don't smoke! It's not too late to stop. Many of the detrimental effects of smoke upon your skin will be improved within a couple of months of your quitting!

BEAUTY ON TAP

Ponce de Leon was on the right track when he went looking for a fountain of youth, but he could have saved himself a great deal of trouble. All along he was sailing on it, drinking it, and (probably only occasionally!) bathing in it. You are even luckier, because the fountain of youth springs right out of your faucet! It's water.

Water is the single most important element for sustaining not only youth and beauty but life itself. You could survive for months without food, but only for days without water. Every cell in the body is bathed in water, and the more you have in your body, the healthier you and your cells will be.

The most expedient way to moisturize your skin is to drink water: A dehydrated body results in dry skin and lackluster hair. You should drink an absolute *minimum* of four glasses a day, and preferably six to eight (that's aside from coffee, tea, soda, juice, or alcohol). Drink even more if the weather is hot, you exercise vigorously, are on a low-calorie diet, or have overindulged in alcohol. You will also get a good supply of water if you eat plenty of fruits and vegetables.

If you have been depriving your skin of the moisture it craves, you will see a *dramatic* difference in its texture within a couple of days of starting to drink more water.

Don't be tempted to skimp on water if you have a tendency to retain fluid, resulting in a puffy face. Paradoxically, drinking water actually *helps* with this problem. Imagine that your body is like a drinking glass. If it is nine-tenths full, it will hold all the water without spilling a drop. But if you put it under a running tap, the water will pour out and will be replaced continually by new water. So if you are not getting enough water, your body will hold on to what it has, but if you drink plenty of fresh water, it will excrete the excess and maintain a proper balance. Drinking water also flushes out sodium and toxins that hold fluids in your body.

In most parts of the country, you can drink water straight from the tap. But if the water in your area is foul-tasting (as it is here in southern California) because of natural mineral deposits or chlorination, install a filtering system or buy drinking water. The type delivered in five-gallon containers is the least expensive, and also can be used for cooking.

Bottled mineral waters have become quite chic in the last few years. There are two kinds: "still" brands, such as Evian, and carbonated types, including Perrier. For drinking in large quantities, the still type may be best because too much carbonation can make you uncomfortably bloated. On the other hand, carbonated water has become perfectly acceptable as a sophisticated alternative to drinking alcohol with a meal, in a bar or at a party.

Develop a taste for room-temperature water; it's better for you than iced. Sip rather than gulp it. And most importantly, don't wait until you are thirsty before you drink: By then, you are already in need of it. If you make a habit of sipping water all day, your skin will thank you by keeping firm, dewy, and young-looking.

Excessive Alcohol—Bad for Your Skin

Like smoking, drinking slows the supply of nourishing blood to your skin, and it inhibits your body's absorption of important vitamins and minerals. This, combined with the diuretic effect drinking has on your body, results in the drinker's skin looking sallow and scaly.

The occasional celebratory binge will have telling but temporary effects. You will probably wake up the morning after with a giant thirst, a puffy face, and circles under your eyes from having had a disturbed night's sleep. Plenty of water, a good meal to replace lost nutrients, and catching up on your rest should put you to rights. However, the more time goes on, the more slowly your skin will recover from these festivities.

To minimize the ravaging effects of a night out and insure rapid "bounce-back," follow these guidelines:

• *Eat before or while you drink.* Your stomach absorbs alcohol twice as fast if it is empty. High-protein, low-fat foods, such as chicken or tuna, give you the best protection. If you have absolutely no time to eat, try the old standby: Drink a glass of milk before you go out.

• *Dilute.* Fill your glass with ice cubes and cut your drink—whether it's spirits or wine—with mineral water. Alternate your alcoholic drinks with sparkling mineral water: Splashed over ice with a twist of lime, it looks enough like a "drink" that people won't pressure you to have another.

• *Rehydrate.* Alcohol acts as a diuretic. Much of the headachy, ill feelings you have during a hangover, and the way they make your face look, are the result of dehydration. You probably won't feel like it, but force yourself to drink several glasses of water before you go to bed.

Heavy, habitual drinking is another story. It can be toxic to your body. Long-term drinking also dilates blood vessels, causing them to break. The alcoholic's face is typically dry, swollen around the eyes, with broken blood vessels on the cheeks and nose. If your drinking has resulted in this type of appearance, your problems are much more than skin deep.

Yo-Yo Weight Gain and Loss Are Bad for Skin

The skin is very accommodating. Every time you gain weight, it stretches to accommodate the fat. When you lose the weight, to a large extent, your skin shrinks back to its original size. But if you put it through this trauma enough times, you will rob it of tone and elasticity.

The answer is to not "yo-yo" up and down the scale. Sometimes maintaining a steady weight, even if it is a few pounds over or under the accepted ideal, is better than constantly striving to reach that goal. A nutritious diet and regular exercise contribute enormously to the beauty of your skin.

Your Skin Reflects Your Emotions

Strain, discontent, disappointment, sulkiness, irascibility—if these are the dominant emotions in your life, over time they will etch themselves on your face in the form of lines. Negative wrinkles—such as frown lines—tend to be much more aging than positive ones, such as laugh lines. Investigate various forms of meditation, or learn a relaxation technique that will help you identify the muscle groups in which you are habitually holding tension. Is it in your forehead, or around the eyes? Are you clamping your jaws shut? By consciously letting go of the strain in your face, you will reduce the chance of developing permanent stress fissures in your skin.

An excellent book to get you started is *The Relaxation Response*, by Dr. Herbert Benson,* Associate Professor of Medicine at the Harvard Medical School and Director of the Hypertension Section of Boston's Beth Israel Hospital. Also find out about the meditation or yoga classes in your community.

---

*Published by William Morrow, 1975.

4. Priming the Canvas

Makeup can make a stunning difference in the way you look—you'll see plenty of evidence of that when you get to our before-and-after makeovers. But cosmetics should enhance your looks, not camouflage them. If you believe makeup can hide neglect, think again! No amount of powder and paint disguises skin that is not moist, smooth, and blemish-free. Beauty begins from the *inside* out, and taking a few simple steps now will give you a facial canvas that's fresh, clear, and youthful.

Consistent care should be your bywords, and that means a sound regimen that normalizes the natural oily/dry condition of your skin, defends it against the environment, and beautifies it. But it must also fit into *your* busy life-style.

If you're anything like our La Costa clients, I think that what you want is: a no-nonsense, streamlined routine . . . products that work . . . remedies for *specific* beauty beefs. It's easier than you might think!

First, zero in on your skin type. No two skins are quite alike, and the clarity, texture, and tone of yours is determined by everything from genetics to environment. But for the sake of simplicity, let's divide skin types into a few broad categories.

SKIN TYPES

Oily. Has a greasy sheen as a result of overactive sebaceous glands. Pores are usually enlarged and coarse-looking: There is a tendency toward blemishes and blackheads. Makeup fades or changes color. That's the bad news. The *good* news is that having a besieged complexion when you were younger might pay back some dividends as you mature; you may wrinkle less quickly and less severely than your dry-skinned friends.

Normal. Perfectly balanced—neither too dry nor too oily. Pores are barely perceptible. Makeup goes on—stays on—beautifully. The danger is that you might take your skin for granted and neglect it, which could spell trouble later on. Actually "normal" skin is something of an idealized nonentity. I've yet to meet a woman who thought her skin was perfectly normal.

Dry. Feels taut and can look flaky. Makeup may cake. Skin is delicate and fine-textured when young—gets many compliments—*but* it wrinkles more quickly than any other types. However, you've probably been rigorous in your caretaking all along, and now Mother Nature needs just a little more of the same help.

Combination. Most women fit in here. Your cheeks are dry, and a T-shaped oily zone runs across your forehead and down the center of your face—you tend to have a shiny nose! Each zone needs separate care.

Sensitive. Affected by hormonal changes, emotions, allergies, weather. Can look red or scaly. Prone to rashes or itching. Any of the other skin types can also be sensitive. Such skin needs professional care and hypoallergenic products. Clarins of Paris, Clinique, and Almay offer an entire range of sensitive-skin-care treatments.

Keep in mind that your category will probably change as you mature. The oily skin that plagued you through your thirties (they lied viciously when they promised that blemishes were only a teenage affliction) starts to become more normal . . . normal and combination skins become dry . . . and dry skin (sorry to say) becomes even drier. Be sensitive to the way your skin is evolving, and revamp your care of it accordingly: It's a good idea to reevaluate your routine every year.

First of all, find a good dermatologist who will be sensitive to your needs. If you're dying to have a few unsightly broken capillaries zapped from your cheeks and a doctor scolds you for being vain and trivial, bid him or her farewell. Some dermatologists are simply more beauty—or cosmetically oriented than others, and it certainly doesn't hurt to ask. Word of mouth from friends is the best way to track down a competent practitioner.

Aside from having a real pro in your corner, you can be your skin's best friend with the well-touted cleanse/tone/moisturize/exfoliate (sloughing off dead cells)/nourish routine. A reminder: It's not what you use as much as *how* you use it in a daily regimen. I see women using the right products *incorrectly* all the time. Treat your adult skin—like your adult hair—with compassion.

YOUR DAILY BEAUTY ROUTINE

There's no room for compromise here. I know you're terribly busy, but (alas, like exercise) the day-to-day efforts are what keep troubles—and the effects of time—at bay. The once-in-a-blue-moon approach to skin is as bad as neglect. You wouldn't think of going through a day without brushing your teeth or tending to your hair, and if you haven't already made skin care a part of your routine, *now* is the time to start. Here are the basic rules:

• You may think that since you weren't "doing anything" as you slept, your skin is already prepared to greet the day. Not true! Your body doesn't stop functioning when you rest; if anything, it plays catch-up with its general maintenance. Sloughed-off dead skin cells mixed with dust are probably clogging your skin. So *cleansing off debris and any residue of night cream or moisturizer is the first order of the day.*

If your skin was oily when you were younger and it still is supple and not too dry, you can wash your face with warm water and soap. The shower is a good place to do it, but don't use *perfumed or deodorant body soaps on your face.* The best soaps for your face are those with the fewest

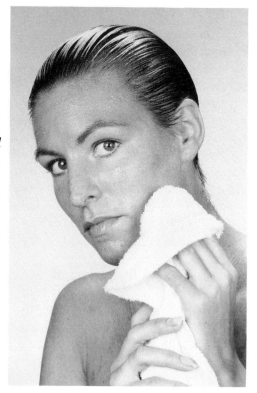

Washing your face, either with or without soap, is a never-to-be-missed first step in the morning.

ingredients that might cause irritation. Dove is particularly mild, and so are Neutrogena, Basis, and Aveeno. Also, many cosmetic houses make superfatted "beauty bars" especially for the face.

If you have dry skin—like most women over forty—be cautious about overwashing. You might wish to forgo soap entirely and simply splash your face well with warm water in the shower. When you wash your hair in the shower, by the way, be sure to rinse the shampoo and conditioner off thoroughly—from face, neck, and shoulders. You're inviting irritation, blocked pores, or flaking if you don't.

Dry your face by patting it gently with a soft, clean towel. Leave it slightly damp, but keep in mind that water must be immediately sealed in with moisturizer or it can actually turn your skin dry as parchment! *Never let water dry directly on your face.*

• Next, smooth moisturizer on to your damp face. Remember to take it down over your neck and throat—areas that are particularly susceptible to showing wrinkles. Now's the time to read your newspaper or eat breakfast, for about fifteen minutes, to allow the moisturizer to *dry* before you apply makeup.

I know it runs contrary to practically everything you've heard, but moisturizer does *not* penetrate the skin. Anything that worked as deeply as some advertisers would have you believe, would require FDA approval. *Water* softens your skin. That's it. The purpose of a moisturizer is to form a barrier that traps whatever water is already present and prevent further evaporation.

You will find any number of moisturizing products available. It's the oil in the lotion that performs the job: The thicker the moisturizer, the higher the oil content. *If your skin is oily, opt for a lighter lotion . . . dry skins need creams.*

For very dry skin, some dermatologists recommend a plain old petroleum jelly such as Vaseline. It's a good humectant (an agent that holds moisture in). And it's cheap, widely available, and nonirritating—you can't ask for a better package than that! If too much of it makes you feel as if you're prepped to swim the English Channel, look for a skin cream that contains petrolatum as the active ingredient. Other ingredients to look for are cocoa butter, mineral oil, and allantoin.

At La Costa we recommend our Collagen Facial Care Line for women who want to retain a *youthful*, supple skin quality. Look for other brands of moisturizer that have collagen as a main ingredient.

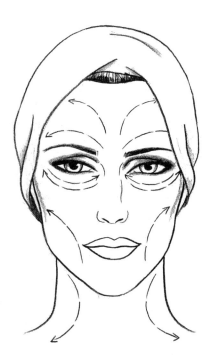

When applying moisturizer, gently massage it in with your fingertips, following the natural lines of the skin on face and neck.

EXERCISING GOOD SKIN SENSE

An active life-style is an excellent means of keeping your skin glowing. Whether you work out in a gym or enjoy the outdoors—swimming, tennis, walking, sports—double the benefits by taking special care of your skin.

• By all means *remove your makeup before exercising.* Otherwise it will run and streak the instant you begin to sweat. Additionally, the makeup might cause irritation and heat rash when your skin warms up.

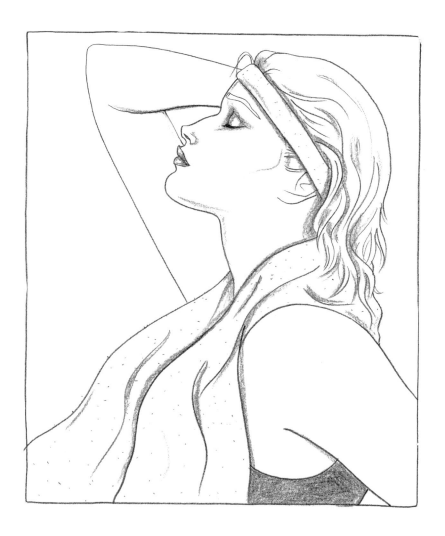

• Wear a terry band around your head to keep sweat from running into your eyes. This will also stop oily scalp perspiration from settling on your face.

• If you are new to the kind of activity that makes you sweat profusely, don't be alarmed if your skin goes through a period of breaking out in pimples and small bumps. That's because your sweat glands are clogged with surface debris, and you may have temporary reaction while it is being washed out. Don't worry—it's a brief inconvenience. After a short time, your skin will be even healthier than before.

• After exercising, thoroughly rinse sweat off your face with lukewarm water, and apply moisturizer while your skin is still damp.

• Don't forget to apply sunscreen, and wear a hat if you are playing an outdoor sport.

• Now you're ready to apply your makeup (which we'll discuss in the next two chapters) if you're running to the commuter train or heading out on the town. But if you're not, why not give your face the day off? Women are so conditioned to "put on their faces" that they miss splendid opportunities for taking a break. Contrary to what many books or magazines might tell you, taking a holiday from makeup is a good idea not because your skin needs to "breathe." It's because every time you do *anything* to your skin—whether it's applying makeup, washing, or removing the day's ravages at night—you are pushing, pulling, and dragging your delicate facial tissue, which exacerbates wrinkling. *Each time you touch your skin, you're weathering it.*

• *At night, don't even think about hitting the pillow before you've removed your makeup and cleansed your face.* I know that romance has a way of making us violate this iron rule. Far be it from me to discourage frolicking; just don't let neglect become a habit.

• Start the cleansing routine with thoroughly washed hands, so that you won't transfer any dirt from your hands to your face.

• *Tackle your eye makeup first.* It can be hard to remove, especially if you are wearing waterproof mascara. A word to the wise: Avoid baby oil or Vaseline to take off your mascara. I know they're convenient, but if you're tried them, you've probably noticed that the slightest errant dab blurs your vision for a while. That's because these products are not water-soluble, and can easily create a film on your eye. Some optometrists have suggested that long-term use could cause a damaging buildup of oil. Avoid the whole messy business by sticking to a nonoily lotion especially made for the job, such as Estée Lauder's Gentle Eye Makeup Remover Liquid.

Unfortunately, since the skin around your eyes is the thinnest on your face and most prone to wrinkling, you're stuck with doing the toughest job on the most delicate area: *Don't* attack as if you're scouring a blueberry stain out of the skin. *Be thorough but gentle.* Apply your eye makeup remover over your eyelids with your fingers in a light, circular motion. For particularly stubborn mascara, apply some remover to a dampened cotton bud and roll it over your lashes until they come clean. Finally, wipe off loosened makeup with a soft white terry washcloth (the dye in colored cloths can irritate your skin) or dampened cotton balls.

Whenever you use cotton balls or buds near your eyes, wet them to dampen down the fibers. Stray fibers can drive your eyes—and you—crazy, causing irritation and redness for hours. Stay away from tissues as well . . . on your eyes *and* face. They're made from wood fibers, and are too rough for your delicate facial skin.

• Now take off the rest of your makeup. I like cleansers, which generally come in the form of lotions and creams, because they're gentle on the skin and don't sap natural oils, as some soaps can. (It takes an oil

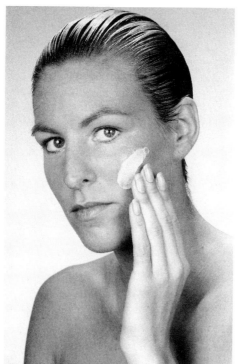

Cleansing cream will remove makeup thoroughly and gently without drying your skin.

to loosen and remove another oil, so if you wear *oil-based* makeup, you need a denser cleansing cream.) Nonsoap cleaners come in several forms. Estée Lauder offers a gel—named, appropriately enough, Thorough Cleansing Gel—Lancôme's Douceur Demaquillante Nutrix is a gentle, tissue-off cream for dry and sensitive skin, and Christian Dior's Hydra-Dior Emulsion Demaquillante is a creamy emulsion with moisturizers.

Either lather up your soap or pour a drop of cleanser into your palm, dab it on your forehead, chin, and cheeks, rub your palms together, and smooth it in. Work it right up to your hairline . . . and don't forget your neck. Gentle massage with your fingertips should do the trick. Don't miss a millimeter—get into the sides of your nose, around your ears, across your top lip. Think of *cleansing* rather than scouring. Wipe off with a warm wash cloth that you've wrung out. Rinse thoroughly by splashing your face with warm water at least ten times; pat dry.

The only true litmus test for choosing a cleanser or soap is by assessing the way it leaves your skin. Is your face taut, dry, or itchy? Does it feel like leather or sandpaper? Switch to a creamier, more emollient product.

• Remove the last vestiges of cleanser with a cotton ball soaked in a toner. (Practically all product lines that carry cleanser also provide a

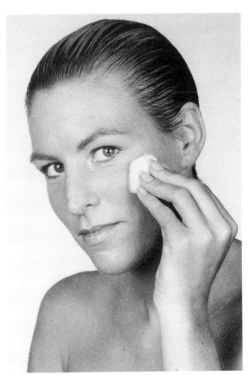

Toner is a stimulating lotion that will remove last vestiges of makeup and cleanser.

compatible toner.) See any traces of makeup on the cotton? It might mean that your cleanser is not efficient enough for your brand of makeup. Try a small-sized bottle of a heavier cream.

Choose a toner designed specifically for your skin—preferably without alcohol. That might be difficult because—surprisingly—even the hypoallergenic brands tend to use alcohol in their toners. A couple of good ones are Biotherm's Tonique Stimulant and Prescriptive's Skin Balancer. Also, check out the cosmetic counter in your local health-food store for plant-based products. Freeman's Aloe Vera skin freshener, for example, contains no alcohol.

• While your face is still dewy, smooth on your night cream. Skim it over your entire face and neck. In the previous chapter, I mentioned the night creams that promote overnight cell renewal—a good bet for mature skins. Bear in mind that a heavy hand is just a waste—your pillowcase probably doesn't need much in the way of a moisturizing job.

• *Then—and don't be tempted to skip this vital step!—carefully dab rich eye cream or oil around your eyes.* Treat these vulnerable, oil-poor areas with special care. Professional tip: Whenever you apply cream to your eye area, put it on with the ring finger of your left hand; it is the digit that exerts the least pressure.

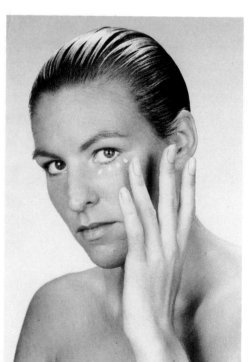

Eye cream will help preserve this delicate area from the ravages of time.

DEALING WITH FACIAL HAIR

After menopause, a drop in your estrogen level can result in an increased growth of hair on your upper lip and chin. It's a common problem, but unsettling if you've never had to deal with it before. Luckily, there are several ways to fight back.

You could seek professional help, in which case your cosmetician might recommend electrolysis, waxing, or bleaching, depending on the growth and the sensitivity of your skin.

If you opt for electrolysis, take care to find a licensed, experienced operator. The hair is "killed" by an electrical current administered to the follicle via a tiny needle. Alternatively, the current is introduced by an electric tweezer, but this method is thought to be less effective. You can buy a home version of an electric tweezer, but incorrect use can lead to infection or scarring, so you would do better to leave hair removal to a professional. The procedure is uncomfortable, and can be expensive. It takes several sessions for the electrolysist to complete the job. But the results are permanent.

I think waxing offers the happiest solution. A professional waxing is quick and effective, and, if done correctly, should be no more painful than having a Band-Aid whisked off. There are kits you can use at home—Sally Hanson's Natural Cold Wax Hair Remover is excellent, and comes with a collagen-enriched desensitizing lotion to apply immediately. Nevertheless, it does sting! If you are too squeamish to do your own waxing ask among your acquaintances to find a salon that uses body-temperature wax, since this is the most effective procedure, and is less potentially damaging to your skin than hot wax. By the way, you're asking for trouble if you submit to a waxing when you are sunburned or if your skin is broken or irritated.

The one disadvantage to waxing is that, although the results last for about a month, you must let the hair grow out substantially before you can have it done again. However, when you wax regularly, the regrowth eventually becomes sparser.

Bleaching also lasts about a month, and can be a good solution if your unwanted hair is not too thick or the growth too heavy. Here too there are home kits that you can use, but because the bleach isn't commercial strength, it sometimes leaves the hair an unattractive yellow—as much a "neon sign" as the original color! There is a temptation to leave the solution on too long when this happens, and that can damage your skin.

Depilatory creams are another home remedy for combating facial hair—although I am not in favor of them. They are caustic, and work by eating away the hair at its root. But since your skin and hair are both largely composed of protein, a cream that is too strong or left on too long will start eating away at the skin. If you must use a depilatory, buy *only* one especially formulated for the face—those for the legs or bikini area are too harsh.

Do not improvise with chemicals, whether they're depilatories or bleaches. Follow the manufacturer's instructions to the letter—including (especially) the one about patch testing the cream for an allergic reaction twenty-four hours before using it on your face.

In most cases, you apply the depilatory generously in the direction of growth, leave it on for about five minutes, and then wipe it off with a warm wash cloth. Rinse thoroughly with lukewarm water.

Immediately soothe the area with a medicated, cooling moisturizer. Both Sally Hanson's and Bikini Bare's facial depilatories come with their own after-care conditioning lotions. Don't use soap or any kind of astringent for a couple of hours after using a depilatory, and, if possible, don't apply makeup until the next day.

A number of women have confessed to me that lopping off the offending hair growth with a razor blade is the easiest solution. I suppose there is no technical reason why that wouldn't work for heavy growth, and it has some exfoliating effect, but I'm against it for several reasons. If you start, you will have to do it every day, because shaving causes blunt-ended hairs that result in bristly stubble and shadow after only a day.

Worse, starting to shave an already lined skin might cause you to cut yourself. This is a time of life when your body is undergoing changes that could be disturbing or confusing. Shaving the face is an intrinsically "masculine" activity, and for that reason alone, I urge you to consider one of the solutions I've listed, which are more suited to feminine facial skin.

YOUR WEEKLY BEAUTY ROUTINE

I firmly believe that *all* women have so many demands made upon them that it's absolutely necessary to set aside just a couple of hours a week on a regular basis for extra pampering. This is never more true than when you start to put up your defenses against Father Time.

Reserving this special time for yourself provides a psychological boost as well as a physical one, because it works wonders for building your self-esteem. So let your family fend for itself, take the phone off the hook, and take a good look at yourself.

• *Check your eyebrows.* Do they need shaping? Your eyebrows can give your face expression and enhance or detract from your eyes and a youthful look.

Don't make the common mistake of tweezing the brows into thin high arches. That creates a hard—not to mention very aging—look. And forget about removing all your brows and drawing in fake ones. Terrible! On the other hand, leave to young girls such as Brooke Shields and Mariel Hemingway the thick, shaggy brows that are currently fashionable. Opt for a neat, trim look instead, especially since eyebrows often do not turn silver when your hair does. An *understated* dark line provides less of a harsh contrast.

Don't waste your time by completely restructuring your brows. Most people have brows that suit their faces. Simply round up the random hairs and refine the shape. Strive for a balanced, natural curve that starts at the inner corner of the eye and extends slightly beyond the outer corner. The highest point of the curve should be just above the outer edge of the iris when you are looking straight ahead at yourself in the mirror.

Before you start work on your brows, clean off your make-up, wash your hands and dip your tweezers in alcohol to sterilize them. Keep your hair off your face with a hair band or towel, and position yourself in a good light, with a magnifying mirror at the ready.

Brush your eyebrows *up* with a cosmetic brush. First tweeze stray hairs growing between the brows. Then shape the brows by tweezing from the underside only. Taper them slightly from the arch to the outer end.

The correct technique is to *tweeze one hair at a time*. Grasp the hair as close to the skin as possible with your tweezers, and remove it with a quick, sharp tug in the direction of the hair growth. After every few hairs, step back and look in the mirror to see how you look full on. Your close perspective could make you a little too tweezer-happy. When you've finished, smooth a little moisturizer over your brows. Once you have attained a flattering shape, you only have to tidy it up on a weekly basis.

• *Another all-important weekly routine should be exfoliation,* which means sloughing off dead skin cells. (Cells are dying all the time.) One of the reasons men's faces seem to age more slowly than women's is that their daily shaving scrapes off the cellular debris. Skin definitely looks silkier and more refined after being retextured by exfoliation. And mature women get added benefits, because as we age, our cells die off in uneven clumps, leaving the skin flaky and dull. But proceed gently, please—your skin is also likely to be dry and sensitive.

Many types of exfoliants are available, in beauty-supply stores, local skin-care salons, or even neighborhood drugstores. They're usually fine facial scrubs, containing an abrasive element, such as crushed apricot kernels or nutshells, in a cream base. Apply them to wet skin and *gently* massage over your face and neck for a few minutes, avoiding the delicate eye area. Rinse off with warm water.

You'll get roughly the same exfoliating effect by using 3-M's Buf-Puf

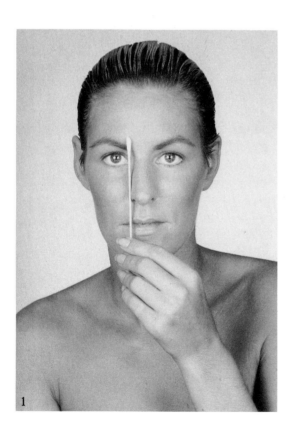

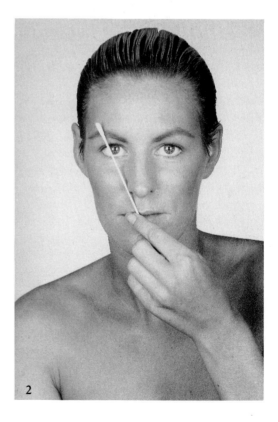

or a similar abrasive sponge. Be sure to use it with a soapy lather or a cleansing cream, and scour your face very gently in a circular motion.

If your face feels tight, inflamed, or irritated after exfoliation, you're either scrubbing too hard or too long *or* using a product that's too gritty. Switch to exfoliating masks—a good tactic for sensitive, mature skins, since they *dissolve* the dead cells rather than *abrade* them.

Apply the mask to a clean face, avoiding the eye area, and leave it on as long as is recommended for the brand you choose—usually about twenty minutes. Exfoliating masks dry to either a peelable film or one you can wash off with warm water.

• *Finish your weekly facial with one of the best instant beauty boosters around: the mask.* (If you've given yourself a "two-in-one" treatment by using an exfoliant mask, you can skip this step.) La Costa patrons rank this "finishing seal" for the skin right up there on the pampering scale with herbal wraps and massages. And it's not only luxurious—it's healthy!

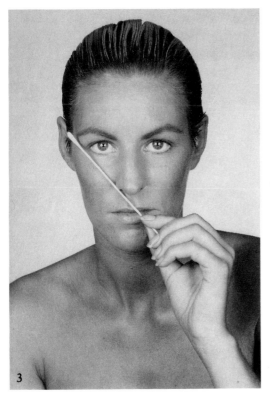

3

Use a cotton swab or long makeup brush held against the side of your nose to help you find the natural shape of your brow. (1) The brow should start in line with the inside corner of your eye. (2) The high point of the arch should be above the outer edge of the iris (where the swab hits your brow when slanted to cross the outer edge of your pupil). (3) The end should be about 1/4 inch beyond the outer corner of your eye (where the swab hits your brow when slanted to cross the outside corner of your eye).

Masks can do all kinds of wonderful things for your skin.

• For stripping surface grease from oily skin, try a mud- or clay-based mask, such as La Costa's Pharmacosta Flower Fresh Clay Masque, Lancôme's Empreinte de Beaute, or Trish McEvoy's Normalizing Clay.

• To hydrate dry skin, look for a creamy mask; for instance, Clarins Cell Extracts Moisturizing Mask, Revlon's Whole Egg Mask, or Dior's Masque Adoucissant.

• Mature, impoverished skin can be nourished with masks rich in minerals, including La Costa's Vitamin EDA Mineral Masque or Anushka's Thermo-Mineral Mask.

• Even tired, drawn skin can get an instant boost from one of the gel masks containing ingredients that promote blood circulation, which accounts for that tingling sensation and rosy glow when you wash it off. Biotherm's Masque Vitalite and Clinique's Beauty Emergency Masque are two good ones.

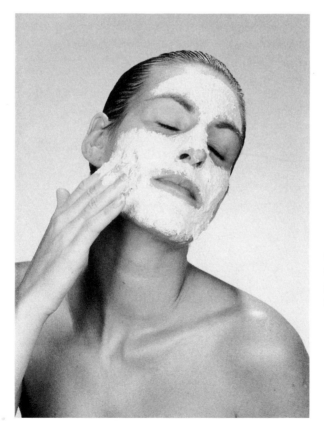

A gentle scrub leaves your skin soft, silky, and glowing; but take care to avoid the delicate eye area.

Apply your mask thinly and evenly to a clean face and neck, leaving a clear circle around your eyes. Put cotton soaked in cold witch hazel or your toner over your eyes to reduce puffiness, and lie down. Relax, with your feet elevated, for twenty minutes, while the mask dries (except for the circulation boosters, which only need to be left on for about three minutes).

Don't be tempted to fill the time by chatting on the phone—you want the mask to dry in a firm way for best results. Besides, why disturb the unadulterated pleasure that comes from doing absolutely nothing?

Once you rouse yourself, remove the mask according to the instructions on the package. Clean off every trace, and then smooth on moisturizer or night cream and leave your face free of makeup for as long as possible. Ideally, you should perform your weekly beauty routine before you go to bed. You and your skin both need time to recover from this much attention!

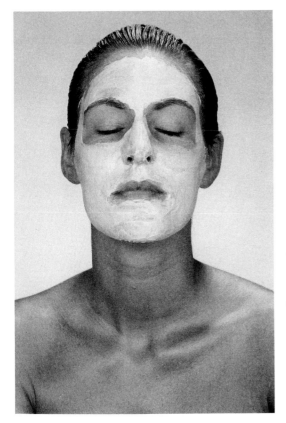

A mask can be the ultimate beauty treatment. Be sure to get one that is right for your skin type.

BEAUTY ON A BUDGET

The list of products you need for a good skin-care regimen can seem daunting, especially when you start looking at price tags. If you are living on a fixed income or simply do not have a budget that will stretch to pricey lotions and potions, you might be tempted to neglect your skin. But good skin care does not have to be an expensive proposition. Here are my tips for achieving beauty on a budget.

• *Become a label reader.* The lower-priced products in a discount drugstore—even in the supermarket!—often have exactly the same ingredients as the higher-priced products sold in department stores. Why pay extra for elaborate packaging and expensive perfumes?

Frankly, not only is the list of ingredients often the same, but many times, the products themselves are identical. I hasten to add that the old adage, "You get what you pay for," still applies somewhat. Most of the good, "name" cosmetic houses have their own laboratories, where they develop products that are worth the price, if you can afford it, because they use higher-quality ingredients.

But many of the mass-market labels simply buy their products from the same factories and charge varying prices. How can you tell? One tip-off is to find the words "distributed by" somewhere on the package in small print.

• *When you are switching to a new product, buy the smallest size first*—even though it goes against every "economy-minded" tip ever written—to make sure you like it *and will not be allergic to it.* Ask the salesperson if he or she has any samples; if not, buy a trial or travel size.

Once you've decided that a product is right for you, go ahead and get the biggest size, for economy. But decant a little at a time into the smaller container for daily use. Repeated exposure to the air and the introduction of bacteria from your hands over a period of months can contaminate your larger supply. Keep your economy bottles and jars tightly capped, in a cool closet or the refrigerator.You can also keep your creams and lotions fresh by using a small spatula, such as a tongue depressor or a small ice-cream spoon, to scoop them out, rather than dipping your fingers into them.

• A number of inexpensive and ultraeffective but "unglamor-ous" products are available at your drugstore. Petroleum jelly can pinch-hit as a makeup remover (don't make a habit of it, though) and as a night cream and lip salve. Try baby oil as an all-over body smoother and a refreshing bath additive. There are different grades of mineral oil and petroleum jelly, so it's worth buying a good, name brand. While you're at it, pick up some witch hazel—the reliable standby for use as a toner.

• Beauty boosters abound at home, but a word of caution: The most up-to-date beauty experts warn that indiscriminate use of foodstuffs on your skin can cause a disaster. Your stomach can cope with the bacteria they contain, but they can cause infections if introduced to the skin by way of cuts or scratches. And if food is too spoiled to eat, why on earth would you want to smear it on your face? Besides, just because something is "natural" doesn't mean you might not be allergic to it!

Here are some simple recipes that will not harm your skin. Since they contain no preservatives, they will not last as long as commercial products, so only make them in small quantities.

Cleansers. Almost any kind of light, water-soluble vegetable oil can be used to remove makeup, but sesame and almond oils are particularly good. Apply with a dampened cotton ball.

Toners. Mix two teaspoons of either cider vinegar or fresh lemon juice in a cup of water, and refrigerate until cold. Use as a freshener—it's even good for dry skin. Slices of freshly cut cucumber rubbed over your face also work well as pick-me-ups. Actually, the cheapest and simplest toner of all is a splash of cold water!

Exfoliants. A very old home remedy is to shake half a tea-spoon of fine table salt into a dollop of rich face cream—Nivea or Oil of Olay are great. Massaged over the face, the salt acts as a mild abrasive, while the cream is the emollient that prevents it from scratching. It's exactly the same principle as the costly exfoliant scrubs. Another homemade facial scrub consists of a couple of tablespoons of oatmeal mixed with a quarter cup of light vegetable oil, such as almond or sesame, until it forms a smooth paste. Massage gently into the skin and rinse thoroughly.

HOW TO GIVE YOURSELF A FACIAL MASSAGE

Massage is at once invigorating and relaxing. Done properly, it can stimulate circulation, boosting the supply of blood and oxygen to your skin's surface. Facial massage can also release tension in the muscles of your forehead and around your eyes and lips—tension that can cause wrinkles. Here's the fabulous La Costa facial massage that we teach to our guests:

When you massage your face, it's important to take care not to drag or pull your skin. That can do more harm than good. You should hardly move the skin at all, but glide over it or press deeply to work the underlying tissue and muscle.

Allow ten to fifteen minutes for a complete face and neck massage—preferably at night, before you go to bed. Make yourself comfortable. You might want to dim the lights and put on some soothing music.

• Start with clean face and hands, and tie back your hair. Using a circular motion with your fingertips, apply a small amount of rich skin cream, light oil, or special facial-massage cream evenly over your skin from neck to hairline. All the time you are massaging, try *consciously* to relax your facial muscles.

• Using your ring and middle fingers, begin your massage on your forehead. With firm but gentle strokes, zig-zag across. Then rotate your fingertips on your temples.

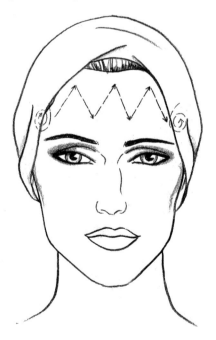

• Using the same fingers, smooth around the eyes, going in toward the nose under the eyes, and out toward the temples on the brow. Use *the lightest possible* touch when massaging around your eyes.

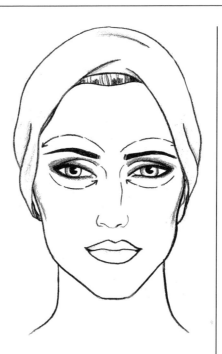

• Now move to your cheeks. Starting with the middle fingers of each hand on your chin, follow your jawline to the base of your ears. Glide fingers to the corners of your nose, using a comfortable degree of pressure. Glide back down to your chin.

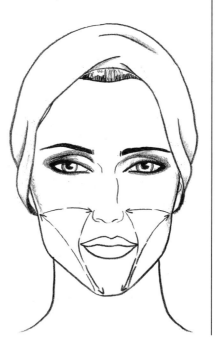

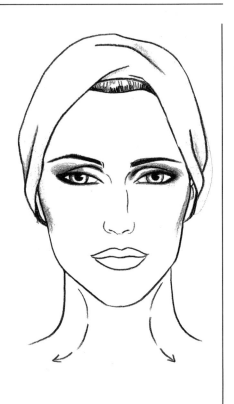

• Using the palms of your hands, massage your neck with a downward motion. Start under your chin and stroke down to your throat.

• If you're not too tired, repeat the massage. When you are done, relax, with your eyes closed, for a few minutes. Then remove cream or oil with a warm, damp facecloth, followed by a few drops of toner on a cotton ball.

Many home facial routines include instructions on "steaming" your face over a bowl of hot water to open pores and deep cleanse. *Don't do it!* Steam is too hot for dry, sensitive, or mature skins, and can cause broken blood vessels on your cheeks. It can also rob your skin of precious moisture. Various steaming treatments may be used during professional facials, but these are done in controlled conditions and under expert supervision.

I highly recommend a professional skin analysis and facial from a licensed cosmetologist whenever your schedule—and budget—allow. Not only is this fabulous for your morale, but a professional perspective might help you head off problems before they become too severe. And what more ideal way to keep abreast of new developments and the best products available for skin care?

If you try the free facial and makeup demonstrations that are offered on the cosmetic floors of department stores, be adamant that the operator use *clean* brushes. Quite frankly, the conditions are not particularly pristine in some instances—the same brushes and sponges are used on countless customers. I am scrupulous about observing the rules of hygiene when I do these "in-store" demonstrations, as are the representatives of most of the reputable cosmetic houses. But, unfortunately, not everyone is.

You should also be aware that salespeople often have a "push" list of products they are trying to sell, and might recommend items that are not really suited to your skin.

That's about all you need to do! Gentle and persistent maintenance will prime your skin to a finish that's soft and youthful. You're all set to pick up your makeup palette and paint yourself into your ideal artistic vision.

PART III

MAKEUP

5. Makeup— Part One: Your Everyday Face

A typical visit to La Costa always includes both a daytime makeup class *and* an evening makeup session. I'll go into special-occasion makeup in the next chapter. In the meantime . . .

Subtle, *believable* daytime beauty is what all women should aim for, but it's especially important for those whose hair and skin have softened in color and texture. *Enhancement, not artifice, is what makeup is about today.* Nothing looks more unattractive than foundation mismatched to skin, harsh stripes of rouge, too-bright or too-pale lipstick, garish eye shadow, or hard-edged eyeliner.

What I like to see least of all is an outdated makeup style. Sometimes you can tell when a woman graduated from college by the way she applies her makeup! So many mature women make the mistake of getting stuck in a beauty rut. It's understandable: They continue using cosmetics in the fashion that prevailed when they thought they were at their best: if their college days were particularly happy . . . if they felt beautiful when they fell in love and married . . . if they had a major success in their careers . . . They have a tendency to stay with the look they had then, almost as if it were a lucky charm.

I'm not suggesting you should be a slave to fashion, throwing out cosmetics every season to restock with the newer colors, or going overboard with wild fads. But by keeping up with the subtleties of makeup

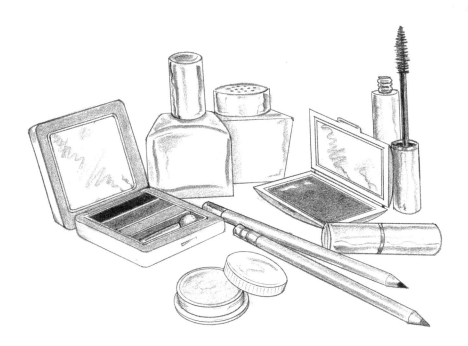

trends, you can add a dimension of fun to your life and be sure of looking *au courant*—that's important if you are in the work force or maintain an active social life.

Staying abreast of trends couldn't be easier—simply read the fashion magazines and scout the department-store cosmetic counters. Better yet, treat yourself to a professional makeup application by a licensed cosmetologist once or twice a year. You'll not only discover what new products and colors are available; you'll also learn how to apply them skillfully.

There is a certain amount of mystique that surrounds makeup application. But I'll demystify it here. Don't be daunted by thinking that you must spend an hour a day resculpting your features. Keep that kind of big-guns glamour for a gala evening event that will take place primarily under artificial light.

In the unforgiving light of day, you want to achieve a soft, flattering effect that camouflages any signs of aging and accentuates your best features. The following step-by-step makeup will do just that. The start-to-finish application won't take more than about ten minutes in the morning, with only a minimum of touching up during the day.

Get off on the right foot (or face) by purchasing the proper makeup tools. They'll make your job much easier, and the results will be absolutely expert-looking.

EQUIPPING YOURSELF FOR BEAUTY

Brushes

The makeup artists at La Costa recommend sable-hair cosmetic brushes: They're soft, natural, and long-lasting—a hard combination to beat! Sable brushes are expensive, but they're durable enough to be a great investment. Buy them in sets or individually. A set often comes with a stand to hold your brushes on your vanity, which also keeps them in good condition and offers easy, at-your-fingertips access to just the right brush at all times. Stand up individually purchased brushes on your vanity in a pretty cup or glass.

Frequent—meaning about every two weeks—washing with mild soap and warm water will keep your brushes in perfect shape. Shake off excess water and allow them to dry naturally.

Here's a sable-collection checklist. Make sure you have the following:

• A flat, slant-tipped brush, about a quarter of an inch across, to blend concealer.

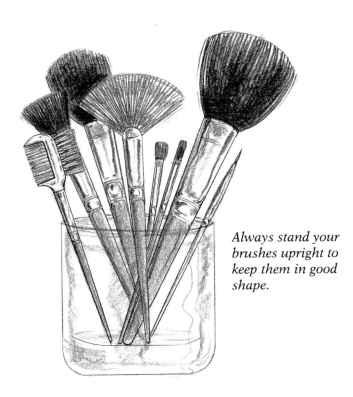

Always stand your brushes upright to keep them in good shape.

- A big, round, fluffy brush for dusting on loose powder.
- A smaller round, fluffy brush for applying blusher.
- A small, pointed-tipped brush for painting on eyeliner.
- A small, soft, slant-tipped brush to apply lip color, whether you use traditional lipstick or color from a pot or compact.
- At least three flat, square-tipped brushes approximately a quarter of an inch across for applying eye color. These are an alternative to the sponge applicators often included with eyeshadows. Throw those sponges out! They absorb oil from your face, and then can streak and muddy your colors. Many women apply eye shadow with their fingertips, but you can contaminate your colors with oil from your hands. And fingers aren't exactly the best precision applicators. Brushes allow you to apply the color smoothly, evenly, and with control.

Other Makeup Tools

Apart from the sable brushes, you will also need:

- A small, stiff brush to shape eyebrows . . . and to sweep powder and foundation out of them. (A small, soft toothbrush works just fine.)
- A tiny comb or (even more effective) a wiry spiral brush to separate your lashes after you have applied mascara.
- Small, natural sea sponges, which are ideal for blending foundation. You'll find them in your drugstore or beauty-supply house for about three dollars. Rinse them out daily under warm running water, and they'll last for years. You can also use wedge-shaped, foam-rubber sponges, which perform quite well but are more difficult to clean. They also start to "crumb" after a couple of washes, and must be thrown away. In the long term, the sea sponges are much more economical.
- Cotton swabs are indispensable for applying foundation, touch-ups, and numerous other makeup chores. Q-Tips make some that are specially for cosmetic purposes, with bigger and softer tips than those of traditional swabs.

Now that you have assembled the tools of the trade, we can start your daytime makeup lesson.

THE TWELVE-POINT DAYTIME MAKEUP APPLICATION

1. Start (always!) with a clean face, toned and moisturized according to your skin type.

2. Concealer is a *must* for most mature women. Just as its name implies, it can hide a multitude of sins.

Concealer comes in a stick or in little compacts of cream. The La Costa makeup artists prefer the cream, because its texture is softer and it's easier to smooth on than the stick. Most of the good cosmetic lines have concealers, but for really hard-to-cover blemishes such as birthmarks, scars, and age spots, try Dermablend Cover Cream. It is a heavy-duty concealer (available from most big department stores) that is greaseless and comes in colors from pale ivory to black skin shades.

Avoid white concealer—it *highlights* rather than diminishes your problem. Instead, choose rose beige if you have cool, blue-based skin, ivory if you have sallow skin with yellow undertones. Concealer should be two shades lighter than your natural skin tone.

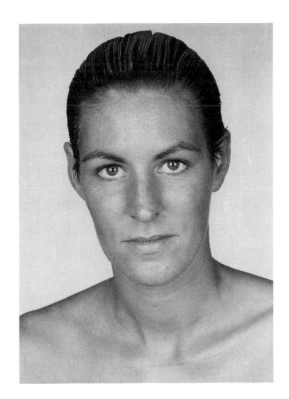

Always start with a fresh, clean face: It provides the perfect canvas for your makeup.

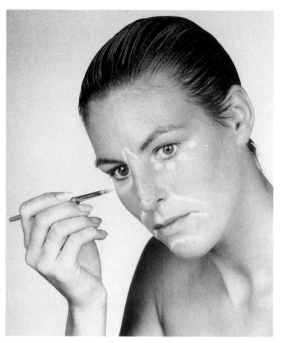

*Carefully blended concealer
can hide lines and discoloration.*

Here is how to apply concealer:

• Dot concealer directly on any dark shadows under your eyes.
• For undereye puffiness, however, apply it in the crease beneath—not directly on—the puffy area.
• Then apply a thin line of concealer in any deep creases you might have around your lips, from nose to mouth, or between brows.
• Finally, dot it on brown spots, broken capillaries, or other areas of discoloration.
• Now use your flat, slant-tipped brush and blend, blend, blend! Smooth the concealer outward, fading it into your skin tone. Remember that the reason for concealer is to even out your skin completely to a clear, one-color canvas. Before applying your foundation, be sure there are no noticeable traces of concealer.

3. Foundation is next. At La Costa, we recommend liquid, water-based foundation for everybody: It gives the most natural cover and is good for all skin types.

When buying foundation, test it on your jawline. Your face and neck are usually two different colors, and your foundation should be midway between those shades, and able to connect face and neck inconspicuously. Color-test foundation every time you buy it, always in daylight. Just because you have used the same color for years does not mean that it is right for you now. Chances are that your skin tone has lightened over the years.

You will also find that you need two different shades, one for winter, and the same color one shade darker for summer. Your suntan foundation simply won't work on winter-pale skin, and vice versa. Between seasons—as your tan builds and fades—blend the two colors by dabbing them separately on your face with swabs and blending with your sponge to get exactly the right shade.

You will find detailed information on color in Chapter 7, but essentially you will be choosing a pinky-beige or rose-colored foundation if your skin tone is cool, with blue undertones, and ivory, peach, or golden colors if your skin has yellow undertones.

One final word on color: *Don't ever attempt to change the natural color of your skin with foundation.* Pancake horror! In the cold light of day, it's terribly artificial and ageing.

Here are the steps for a flawless foundation finish!

• Rinse your sea sponge in water, and squeeze it out thoroughly in a towel. A sponge that's too wet will take off your concealer and streak your foundation; slightly moist, it will give you an even, natural cover.
• Dip a cotton swab into your liquid foundation and dab it on your forehead, cheeks, chin, and nose. Doing it this way avoids contami-

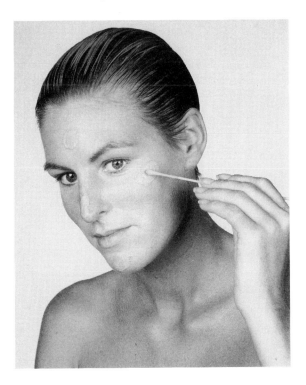

Apply foundation with a clean cotton swab.

nating foundation with the oil and dirt from your hands. If you are mixing two colors, dab them directly on to your face with two separate swabs, and blend them on your skin.

• Now use your damp sea sponge to blend in your foundation. Take it up to your hairline and just over the curve of your jaw. Do not take foundation down your throat, and avoid your eyelids, so that they are clean for your eye makeup.

4. Blusher—it's indispensable, but keep it to a minimum and blend it well. "Slashes" of color are too severe for you. Use it to warm your face and to give it a natural glow.

Choose a color that blends with your skin tone: clear-blue/pink and dusty-rose shades for skin with blue undertones, peach and tawny shades for skin with yellow undertones. If your hair is completely silver or very light, choose from the pale end of the spectrum. Avoid shimmery or glossy blushers. They reflect light, and can emphasize lines. Opt instead for soft, matte versions of your chosen color.

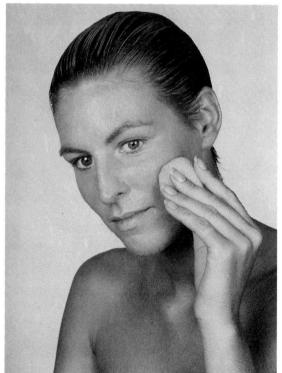

A damp sea sponge blends your foundation to a flawless finish.

Which blush to choose—cream or pressed powder? Both are easy to apply, but I recommend cream for dry skin, and powder for oily skin (the oil on your skin dilutes the color in cream blusher, so that it fades during the course of the day). Professionals at La Costa actually use both—cream first, then a dusting of powder blush to set the color.

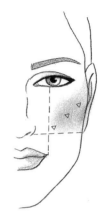

To apply cream blush:

• Dab three dots of color on each cheekbone (see illustration).
• Using your fingertips, gently blend up and outward, toward your temples. Blend with a "patting" motion, rather than smoothing it in.

To apply powder blush:

• Sweep your sable brush *once* across the pressed powder. That's all the color you'll need.

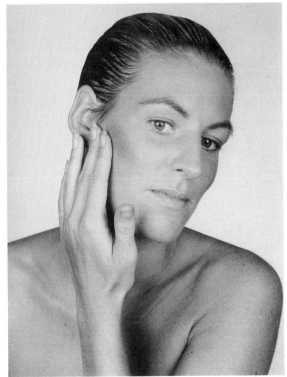

Blend cream blush by dabbing or patting with your fingertips.

• Tap the brush on your hand to knock off the surplus.
• Buff your cheekbones with the brush until the color is well blended—you should not see any demarcation lines.

Don't take blush lower than the imaginary line that extends from the tip of your nose to the side of your face, and no further in toward the center of your face than the middle of your eye. Our diagram shows you exactly where to place it.

Give a pale face a glow by *sparingly* dusting your blusher on nose, chin, and temples. It does more than anything to make you look and feel alive!

5. Face powder is optional. You get a more natural look for daytime by giving it a miss. Women who have facial lines might discover that powder can settle in creases, drawing attention to them. But if your skin tends toward oiliness—or if you want a more polished look—by all means finish your face with translucent, loose powder that comes in a shaker-top bottle.

Shake a little into the palm of your hand; then fluff it all over your face—except on your eyelids—with your largest sable brush. As with powder blush, buff off the excess. The effect should be matte, not caked.

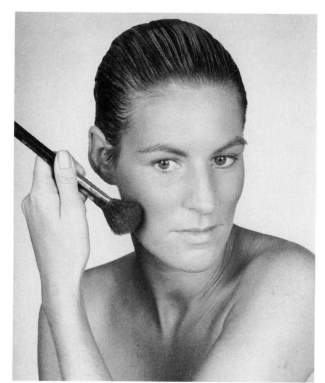

Use a large brush to fluff loose powder on, then to buff it well.

6. Eyebrows are always either too much or too little, we neglect them *or* we subject them to all sorts of tweezing and unnatural abuse. And that's a shame, because they're one of the most important features on your face. What else does as much to make you appear sad, happy, angry, or surprised? Something that powerful deserves special attention. I talked about shaping eyebrows in the previous chapter; now here are some makeup guidelines.

- Use your small, stiff brush to remove foundation and powder from your brows.
- Now brush them into shape: sweep hairs up and out toward your temples, brush the outer half down from the top.
- If they need some extra definition or if their shape has some irregularities, fill them in with short, feathery strokes from well-sharpened eyebrow pencils.

   Use a color close to that of your own hair, or even a little lighter. The most natural effect can be achieved by mixing two colors, such as blond and taupe, or light and medium gray. Never use black—with your silver hair, it will look much too harsh.

- Brush lightly again to blend colors. Unruly brows can be tamed by putting a tiny dab of hair mousse on the brush.

7. No other makeup comes in as many forms—not to mention colors—as eye shadow. You'll find it in powders, creams, gels, pencils, and crayons. Mature women should steer clear of creams and gels—they melt into creases and accentuate lines. Forgo pencils and crayons, too—applying them drags and pulls the delicate skin around your eyes. A better bet—pressed powder, the *best* bet—watercolors. That's all we use at La Costa.

Because watercolors are applied with a wet brush, you can regulate the intensity of the eye shadow, from a thin, subtle wash to a concentration of color. You can also compound the effect by blending different shades. Best of all, watercolors last much longer without fading, creasing, or smudging.

La Costa has a full range of watercolor eye shadows in its catalog. But many of our clients have reported excellent results simply by applying their pressed-powder shadows with a wet brush, thus transforming them into watercolors. It's worth a little experimenting!

I recommend soft, smoky tones for silver-haired women . . . but don't think that I'm shortchanging you, because although you should shun the pastels, "icy" pales, and brilliant, jewellike shades, there's still an infinite palette available in your range. As with blush, forgo shimmery shadows (for daytime, at least) in favor of matte colors.

A word of warning before we discuss particular shades: Please don't make the mistake of matching your eye shadow to your clothes. That's an outdated beauty concept! Instead, color-key your eye shadow to your eyes. This is not to say that you should use eyeshadows that are the *same* color as your eyes—merely ones that *bring out* your baby blues or chestnut browns.

Blue and gray eyes will be most enhanced by taupe, slate, navy blue, and smoky lavender. Highlight under the brow bone with rose beige; soft, dusky pink, or pale silvery gray.

Green and hazel eyes are flattered by olive green, deep plum, and spicy browns such as paprika; highlight with peach, creamy-white, or oyster.

Brown-eyed women are lucky because they can wear the whole range of hazy, earth tones, ranging from rust to camel, copper, and moss. Ivory makes a pretty highlighter.

GLAMOUR IN GLASSES

Women who wear glasses often complain to me that it's almost impossible to apply eye makeup—they can't see clearly enough without their glasses! This causes most of them not even to bother, even though *eyes behind lenses need more color and definition than others.* Don't neglect yourself, because your glasses frames actually *draw* attention to your eyes.

Keep your glasses at hand and put them on to check at every stage. Also, ask your optician about glasses with lenses that flip up and down. These will allow you to see clearly one eye at a time. While you're at it, invest in a large magnifying mirror, the type with lights around the edge, available in most drug and department stores.

If you're farsighted, keep in mind that your lenses *magnify* both your eyes and your eye makeup. Eye shadow should be a *subtle* blend of colors neatly applied. Be sure your eyelashes are not clumped together, and keep your eyebrows neatly tweezed.

Glasses for nearsightedness make your eyes look smaller. Makeup can work wonders in emphasizing them, but don't make the mistake of using overbright colors. Stick to the smoky

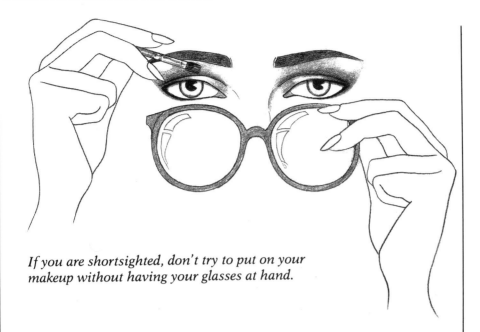

*If you are shortsighted, don't try to put on your
makeup without having your glasses at hand.*

shades, but don't be shy about applying them a little more
intensely than normal, particularly when it comes to the contour line.

Here are some other general tips.

• Lenses of any kind have a tendency to darken the eye area.
Cover those dark circles under your eyes meticulously with
concealer and foundation.

• Be careful not to let your glasses dominate your face!
Lipstick can act as a balancer. Pale lip colors will cause your
lower face to fade away, so stick to sheer, clear washes of bright
color.

• When it comes to eyeglass frames, silver-haired women
should shun dark colors. Tortoiseshell, black, bright-colored
plastic, and decorated or patterned frames are much too overpowering for your delicate coloring. Stick to thin gold or silver
rims, clear or light-colored plastic frames, or consider rimless
styles.

• If you choose to wear tinted lenses, they should not contain
more than 5 percent color. The tint should tone with, or complement, your eye color. Be careful with brown lenses, though,
they sometimes have a nasty way of making your eyes look
tired.

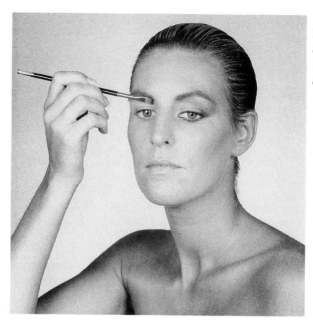

There is no mystery to applying perfect eye makeup if you have the right tools and a little know-how.

Eye-shadow application is simple if you follow these guidelines;

• First, apply your highlighter shade—such as rose beige or soft ivory—over your entire lid, from brow to lash line. Your other colors now have a base, *and* your highlighter is in place under the brow line.

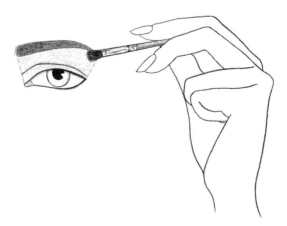

• Add contour with a darker *but neutral* color, such as taupe or gray. This line should not be in the crease of the lid, but *above it*. At the outer corner of the lid, bring the color down to the lash line.

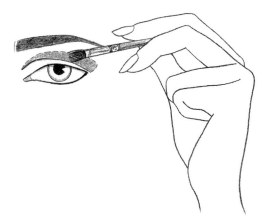

• Now add some pizzazz with a wedge of an accent color at the outer corner. Then take a fine line of the accent color along the lower lash line. This accent color should be brighter than, but tone with, your contour color.

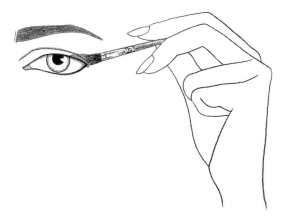

• Finally, smudge all the colors together with a damp (not wet) brush. Your eye shadow should be blended so subtly that you can barely identify any of the individual colors.

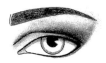

EYE LINER FOR LIFE

One of the most revolutionary breakthroughs in the makeup world in recent years has been the introduction of permanent eye liner. Natural pigment is surgically implanted into the dermis of the eyelids. The technique is akin to tattooing. But don't worry about feeling like a seaman on leave, the equipment used for eye lining is much finer than what's used to burn *Mom* on a burly chest, and the microscopic needle penetrates no more than one millimeter into the skin.

The needle introduces micro-dots of color along the base of the lash line and between the lashes, upper and lower. You can choose varying intensities of black and brown shades, and the line can be as thick or as thin as you like. You can then apply your daily eye-shadow colors over the top of the line.

What are the advantages of permanent eye liner? It's great for women who have allergies and are not able to wear conventional eye makeup. Older women who find it difficult to apply eye liner because their hands are becoming less steady are possible candidates, as are women who wear glasses and can't see clearly enough to apply eye makeup. Active women who play sports or swim also find it practical.

Dermatologists, plastic surgeons, and ophthalmic surgeons perform the procedure, and in most parts of the country it costs about a thousand dollars. The procedure must be done in an operating room, although it only takes about an hour. The process leaves a crusty surface that takes about a week to heal. If you decide to have the prodecure done, find an *experienced* practitioner (referrals are, once again, your best bet for finding someone reputable).

To date, only one potential problem has arisen. Some women have had allergic reactions to some of the pigments. Apart from that, the big disadvantage, of course, is that the effect is permanent. If you don't like it, you are still stuck with it.

Silver-haired women should proceed with caution! A line that is dark or thick can look too heavy. And as your hair gets progressively lighter, the eye line might look more and more out of sync. Opt for a fine line in gray or light brown. Be sure that the upper line does not extend beyond your natural lash line at the outer corners, and the lower line extends no more than three-quarters of the way from outer to inner corners.

"Permanent" eyeliner can be applied in varying intensities: thin, medium, or thick.

8. You may prefer to dispense with eye liner entirely. I think it adds a nice definition and accent to eyes. You might simply use a dark shade of eye shadow, or choose a *water color* eye liner in gray or brown—never black, it's simply too harsh. Using your eye-liner brush, paint a fine line at the lashes on your upper lid, from inner to outer corner. *Don't* extend it beyond the natural line of your eyes. On the lower lid, paint the line only on the outer half. Then, before the liner has totally dried, use a damp cotton swab to blur the lines gently.

9. Mascara adds the finishing touch to your eyes. Many women have returned to the old-fashioned cake type, which offers control in terms of how lightly or darkly it can be applied. Dampen the brush and rub it gently over the cake; then stroke it onto your lashes. Add successive coats until you have achieved the desired look. Never, *never* wet your mascara brush with saliva: It contains bacteria that can infect your eyes. Wash the brush after every application to prevent dried mascara from clumping on the brush.

Wand mascara is generally quicker and more convenient to use. A professional tip: There is no need to pump your brush in and out of the container in order to get mascara on it. This forces air into the tube, which prematurely dries out your mascara. Twirl the wand in the tube a couple of times—you'll get all the mascara you need.

Apply mascara to your upper lashes first. Tilt your head back and look down as you sweep the mascara brush from close to the lid to the tips of your lashes. Then do your lower lashes by tilting your head down and looking up. A couple of light coats are better than one thick one. Separate lashes with your spiral brush or lash comb between coats.

While waterproof mascara is also smudge-proof and impervious to floods, hurricanes, and aerobics classes, it is difficult to remove, and requires much rubbing of delicate eye skin. I recommend the water-removable type.

Some brands contain particles to build up lash thickness, but they tend to flake off and leave little spots on your cheeks. Worse, they can irritate or scratch your eyes, especially if you're a contact-lens wearer. If any of this happens to you, *don't* grin and bear it. Switch brands!

Silver-haired women should avoid black mascara and such "unnatural" colors as purple or blue for daytime. Opt for charcoal, brown-black, or golden brown.

10. Even if you've never used a lip pencil before, give it a whirl. You'll be surprised at how much more polished you look. In any event, this is a vital makeup step for women who have tiny lines around their mouths, as it prevents lipstick from "bleeding."

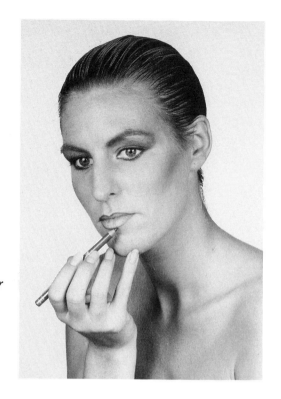

Outline your top lip first, then your bottom lip, with a well-sharpened pencil.

For best results, your lip pencil should be soft, waxy, and *always* sharpened to a point. Let me warn you in advance: Sharpening lip pencils can be infuriating. Because they're so waxy, they usually break in the sharpener just as you are achieving a good point. A never-fail (well, almost never) La Costa tip: Put your pencil in the freezer for an hour before attempting to sharpen it, but let the tip soften again before using the pencil.

Outline your top lip first, using short, even strokes, and then do the bottom lip. If your hands tend to be unsteady, rest your fingers on your chin while drawing your lip line.

To minimize thick lips, draw slightly *inside* the natural lip line. Give a fuller look to thin lips by drawing just *outside* it, although this might not be possible if you have vertical lines around your mouth. In that case, make your lips look fuller by avoiding dark shades in favor of softer, slightly shimmery lipsticks.

Too-obvious lip lining is arguably the biggest makeup blunder a woman can commit. Keep it imperceptible and blended with your lipstick—*defined but subtle.*

11. Lip color comes in little compacts as well as the familiar stick form. If lip color tends to "bleed" on you, choose the firmer-textured sticks. When bleeding is a serious problem, choose one of the products on the market today that you apply under lipstick to "fix" it. Elizabeth Arden has one, appropriately called Lip Fix. There are also a number of brands of lipstick especially formulated to combat bleeding: Estée Lauder's Featherproof Lipstick and Coty's Luminescent Lipstick are two fail-safe ones.

For daytime, strike a balance between matte and shiny textures, and pick colors in the midrange between pale and strong. I don't think pastel colors with white or chalky undertones flatter mature women—too washed out!—and while intense colors look sophisticated on you, reserve them for your big nights out. Aim for a slick of clear, defining, but not overpowering color, such as rose or coral.

Apply lip color with your lip brush. Keep the area relaxed—no open mouth or smile. Precisely fill inside the liner, and blend carefully. Blot with a tissue.

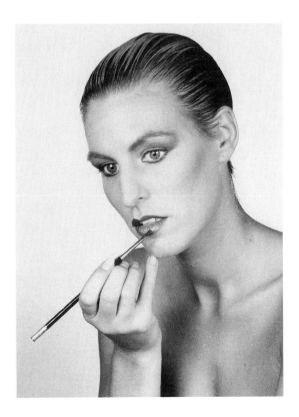

Always apply lip color with a clean, slanted brush.

12. Tend to your hair and finish dressing—and now take a final look at yourself in the mirror. Do you need another lick of color on your cheeks? A dusting of face powder if your facial oil has already broken through? Are your eye colors cleanly blended? Is the overall look natural, sophisticated, warm? Once your makeup's impeccable: *Forget about it!* You'll need to reapply your lipstick after lunch, but that should do it. You're ready to step out and greet the day.

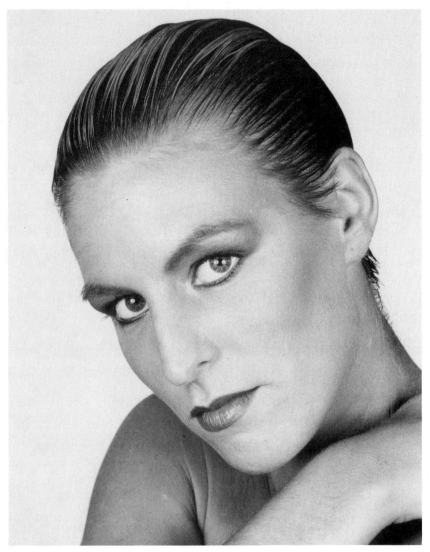

Correctly applied makeup can create a more dazzling you by enhancing the real *you.*

6. Makeup— Part Two: Nighttime Dazzle

Silver-haired women can indulge in the kind of drop-dead glamour that no twenty-year-old can carry off. I've seen plenty of young girls beautifully done up, but I'm truly bowled over by a woman who's stunning, self-assured, and very much *herself*—something that only comes with maturity. With a strong sense of self and the confidence that comes with time, a silver-haired woman can look coolly elegant, sizzlingly sophisticated, when she pulls out all the stops for a special occasion.

Don't try to make your daytime makeup work at night, because artificial light strips color from both your face and makeup. Be daring! After dark, you're allowed a flagrant flouting of some of the makeup rules: Add a touch of shimmer . . . the opulence of rich color . . . a bold bright effect. Go ahead and dazzle.

FACES AFTER DARK

Now's the time to bring out the big guns of contouring and highlighting. These techniques can be effective, but require practice. Don't be tempted to try face sculpting for the first time right before a special occasion. Sorry—it's more difficult for mature women to get away with the sloppiness or extremes.

Bear in mind that the word *cosmetic* derives from the Greek *kosmetos,* which means "order and harmony." It's a good rule: Makeup artistry should create order and harmony. So take some time to experiment with and become adroit in these techniques, which only require a few minutes more than putting on your basic makeup: High impact doesn't have to mean high effort.

The object of sculpting? To soften any angular lines, to slim or downplay broad areas and emphasize others, and to mold bone structure where yours is not apparent.

Here are the elements:

• A cream highlighter in a flesh tone two shades lighter than your own. (Don't confuse highlighter with your concealer. The latter is usually a creamy consistency made for covering flaws. Highlighter is a lighter liquid—more like your foundation—that contains a little shimmer.) Light tones *reflect* light, so you will be using your highlighter to bring certain features into prominence. But avoid white, which looks unnatural. Pat the highlighter over your foundation (according to the following instructions) before you dust with translucent powder.

• A contour powder a couple of shades darker than your skin tone, and a brush—such as your blusher brush—to apply it. You could use a matte tone of blush in a color darker than your usual one. The dark color slims and defines. It should be applied when you also apply your regular powder blush. (Your blusher also will be used in the face-shaping process.)

Everyone's face is a different shape, making it almost impossible for us to fit *exactly* into some formula of diamond, round, heart-shaped, and so on. But, as with skin types, there are broad categories—in this case five basic structures—that cover most of the bases. You'll know from years of staring at your face in the mirror what are the broadest and narrowest parts of it, and which irregularities you would like to correct.

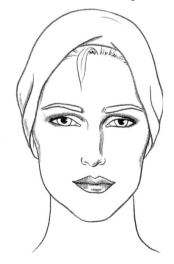

• *Oval is the classic and ideal shape.* If you are lucky enough to have a face that is neither too long nor too broad, don't even worry about sculpting it. Apart from simply enhancing it with color, the only other thing you might try is emphasizing your cheekbones. A La Costa tip for bringing out your cheeks at night: Dust a *very* slightly iridescent powder—you could use a pearly ivory eye shadow—on the top edge of your cheekbones. Blend it softly into your blush. The effect should be soft and dewy—not shiny.

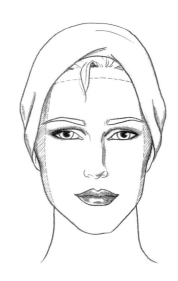

• *A round face has width at the cheeks and, usually, a narrow forehead.* Apply a band of highlighter about an inch wide across the top of your head at your hairline, and blend in thoroughly.

Shade with contour around your hairline, from the temples to below the corner of your mouth. Do not apply shade on the tip of your chin. When blending, carry the contour well into the widest part of your cheeks. Your blusher should be applied in a *narrow* band. If you make it too wide at the outer edge, it will broaden your face further.

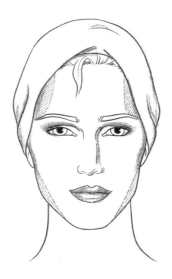

• *A square or rectangular face has angular lines at the forehead and jawline.* Soften them with shading at the outside corners of your temples and jaw. Be careful when applying blusher not to take it up higher than your natural cheekbone.

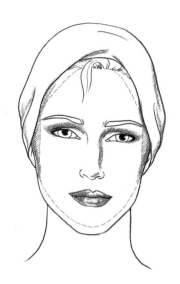

• *A diamond-shaped face has wide cheeks, a pointed chin, and a high forehead.* Apply highlighter at the outside edge of your forehead and along the jawline and chin. Your shading should be blended from where highlighting stops, just above your brow, and extend to below your cheekbone along your hairline.

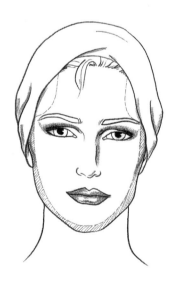

• *A pear-shaped face is jowly, or bottom-heavy.* Blend in a little highlighter at your temple area. Shade all around the outside of your face, from eye level to eye level. Your blusher can sweep up and out toward your temples.

Apart from correcting facial shape, you can also sculpt individual features on your face. More refined shaping and shading requires special expertise. Don't be put off, but do practice until you are proficient at applying your face paints in such a way that only *you* know they are there.

• You can create cheekbones on the chubbiest of faces with a little makeup artistry. Apply contour powder in the hollow of your cheeks, right below your cheekbones—find the correct place by sucking in your cheeks. As with blush, contour should come no further into the middle of your face than the center of your eyes.

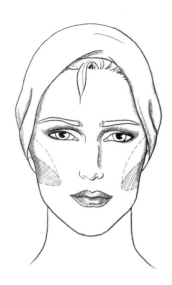

Then apply your blush, which should be a lighter shade, in the usual place on your cheekbones. Buff the two together with a brush until they are well blended. There should be no demarcation line between the two colors.

• I wish I had a quarter for every woman who's complained about her nose! It causes more consternation than any other facial feature.

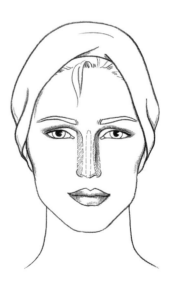

A broad nose can be slimmed by shading on the sides and applying highlighter in a stripe down the center. Reverse the process for a thin nose. As always: Blend well.

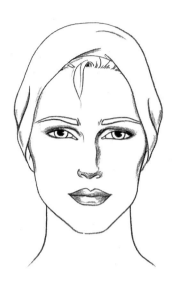

• As the years go by, our noses tend to lengthen slightly. To give the illusion of shorter nose, use your contour powder—easy does it—on the underside of your nose between the nostrils.

• Play down a double chin by dabbing highlighter on the point of the chin and contouring just under the jawline from ear to ear and down the throat. Be extra careful to wield your brush and fade the colors into your skin tone—otherwise you'll look as if you have a dirty neck!

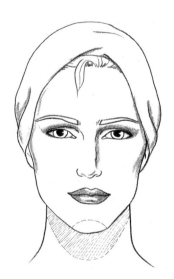

EYES GO GLAMOROUS AFTER DARK

I can tell a lot about a woman just by looking at her eyes. And with time, eyes only get *more* beautiful . . . they truly reflect the wisdom and experience that comes with maturity. It's worth learning a few tricks to show them off:

• *Use a softly iridescent powder to highlight your brow bone at night.* Steer clear of extremely pearlized shadows, which can accentuate crepiness. When it comes to color, pass on white—it's way too harsh. Ivory, peach, rose, or lavender will give you a glow that opens up your eyes.

• *A touch of gold—very much in vogue—can equal a touch of class.* Judiciously applied, it adds luminosity to a nighttime makeup. In fact, this Midas touch can instantly turn a day look into evening drama! Many cosmetic companies have gold-toned lipsticks, eye shadows, and even mascaras in their palettes. A casual sweep *over the top* of your existing colors is enough. A haze of gold on your brow bone balanced by a smudged dot in the center of your lips will be all you need. Stunning! (But—forgive me for sounding like a broken record—*restraint* is the key.)

• *Silver, to match your hair, can be another showstopper.* Confine its use to your eyes. Blend a little on the inner corners of your eyelids for a bright-eyed, wide-awake look.

• *Apply your contour eye color a little more intensely than usual.* Also, be bolder with your accent color at night, but don't give in to brilliant, jewellike colors. They look vulgar—too much like a crayon box—on mature women. Go for something different, subtle, *deep;* like say, burgundy, bronze, or pine.

• *Eye liner can stand to be more defined at night.* It can rim your entire upper and lower lids. Additionally, you can use a soft, smudgy pencil in the same color as your liner to draw a line in the lower *inner* lid above your lashes. It is an exotic look that makes the whites of your eyes very bright. But your eyes will look smaller, so use this tactic at your discretion.

• *Women who are only partially silver or have dark, iron gray hair can try black mascara in the evening.* But if your hair is very light, stick to brown or charcoal—or be adventurous by applying colored mascara. I love seeing this softly exotic note as a delicate accent to an evening makeup. Experiment with blue or violet—or be *really* bold with deep red, yellow, or turquoise. Just make sure your mascara blends with your eye shadow—too much contrast looks garish. Midnight blue, for example, looks good with all the cool blues, grays, and lavenders.

PUTTIN' ON THE GLITZ

I'm adamant about the importance of jewelry in completing a glamorous look. It's not exactly makeup, but the jewelry you wear close to your face—namely earrings and necklaces—adds the final touch, and should harmonize with the rest of your look. I asked Pepi, a Beverly Hills jeweler whose designs are nationally renowned, for her jewelry tips—*especially* since Pepi is a striking silver-head herself! She was happy to share the following tips with you:

• Mature women look just smashing in everything from classic pearls to sparkling diamonds. Many of the colored stones—

Wearing one or two carefully chosen pieces of jewelry is far more elegant than piling on everything you own.

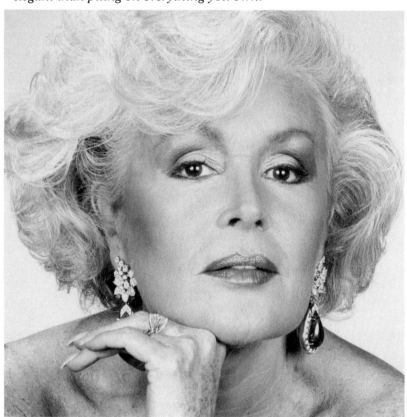

emeralds, rubies, topaz—are set off beautifully by silver hair. When it comes to precious metals, silver, platinum, and white gold will look *particularly* stunning on you. Although gold, of course, looks wonderful on anyone, you might find that brushed gold compliments your coloring more than shiny gold.

• Don't wear everything at once. You probably have collected some well-loved pieces of jewelry by now, and there is a temptation to want to show it off on a dress-up occasion. This approach is not only vulgar; it detracts from the beauty of the individual pieces—and from you! You should wear your jewelry, not the other way around. Showcasing one or two pieces at a time is far more elegant and tasteful.

• Occasionally, jewelry with heavy or ornate settings might begin to appear overwhelming with your softer coloring. Let your own judgment guide you. One suggestion: Have your stones reset in a more delicate surrounding.

• There's nothing wrong with costume jewelry; in fact, it's very fashionable right now. But you have to be a little more choosy than before your hair turned silver. Good taste is all-important. Avoid faddy, gaudy baubles . . . anything made from plastic, paper, bits of lace, and sequins . . . fake gold chains—they always look cheap.

Perfectly acceptable, however, are frankly *faux* high-fashion pieces—chunky colored stones, good-quality rhinestones, giant "pearls"—that complement your clothes and personal style.

Jewelry draws attention to itself, so bear the following in mind:

• Choker-style necklaces make your neck look shorter. They will also call attention to a lined or crepy neck. Opera- or matinee-length strings of pearls or chains are often more flattering.

• Long, dangling earrings lengthen your face—ideal if you have a broad face or short neck, *not* so ideal if you have a long or downward-drooping face.

• Chunky, stud-style earrings do just the opposite. They are perfect for adding width to a long face.

• If you have worn long or heavy earrings for years and years, you might have stretched your earlobes, and dangling, pierced earrings could look painful (and unattractive) now. Opt for clip-on styles that camouflage your lobes.

• *Add fullness to very pale or sparse eyelashes.* I'm all in favor of false lashes. Go for light, evenly spaced lashes made from natural hair that adhere as closely to your own lash line as possible. If you have a very steady hand, try cutting the lashes into small clumps and sticking them on individually. Taper them at the outer and inner corners of your eyes, just as your own lashes do. Make certain they're secure by pressing them firmly into place. The final step: Stroke mascara on to both your natural and false lashes to blend them together.

SHEDDING SOME LIGHT ON THE SUBJECT

Why go to all the trouble of glamorous makeup, only to have the lighting ruin it in one, glaring stroke? Are you going to be seen in fluorescent light? Electric light? Or (best of all!) candle-light? Make yourself up, or at least check yourself out, in the same type of lighting that you will be seen in.

Alas—most artificial forms of light are very unflattering to the skin. Here are some remedies.

Electric table lamps tend to make your face look flat. Be a little more heavy-handed with your contouring.
Overhead electric lights cast shadows that can be aging. Use concealer skillfully.
Fluorescents are the most merciless of all. They'll drain color, especially pink tones. Compensate by applying extra blush and deeper-color lipstick.

When you don't know what lighting awaits you or if you don't have the wherewithal to recreate it, at least give yourself a fighting chance of looking good by applying your makeup in the *best* available (meaning strong but unglaring) light.

Why not treat yourself to a professional makeup mirror in your bedroom or bathroom? You've seen them in movies about the theater—the star always has one in her dressing room. They have a strip of frosted lightbulbs evenly spaced across the top and down each side. Buy these strips of lights at a good hardware store, or ask a handyman to build one for you. And you should also have a large hand mirror so you can check your profiles and the back of your hair.

SECRETS OF EYE SHAPING

On those extraspecial occasions, particular attention to eye shaping can help to customize and sculpt your look.

• *Small Eyes.* Cover your whole lid, from lash line to brow, with a light, shimmery shadow to open up the space. Sweep your contour and accent colors slightly up and out at the outer corners. Apply your upper and lower eye liner only on the outer two-thirds of your eye. Use a soft white pencil to line the lower inner lid. *Never* use a dark inner liner—it will make your eyes look even smaller. If you have short or straight eyelashes, use an eyelash crimper. Curling the lashes upward is an added eye-opener.

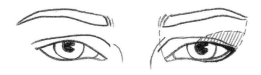

• *Bulging Eyes.* Stay away from light-reflecting (bright and glossy) eye shadows. Your base and highlighter should be matte and neutral—why not see if your powder blush works? Instead of emphasizing the crease, apply a smoky or earth-tone shadow over the eyelid, and blend it upward until it fades away. Complete the look with a charcoal or dark brown pencil on the inner lower eyelid.

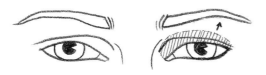

• *Close-Set Eyes.* Apply a light-colored or faintly iridescent shadow on the inner corners and blend it right up to the sides of your nose. Wing your accent color up at the outer corners almost to the eyebrows. As with small eyes, concentrate your liner on the outer two-thirds of your top and bottom lids.

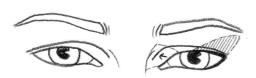

• *Wide-Set Eyes.* Reverse the close-set principles by applying your darker color on the inner corners of your lids and blending it softly toward the center. Your upper and lower eye liner should start at the inner corner and maintain the same width, or even taper, at the outer corner.

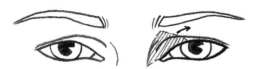

• *Hooded Eyes or Overhanging Brows.* Even if you don't start out in life with overhanging brows, they could sneak up on you in time. Bushy brows make the problem worse. Take special care to tweeze your eyebrows neatly from the undersides and brush upward. Avoid using shiny or overly pale colors on your brow bone. Choose deep contour color for your eyes, and blend it upward toward your brows to diminish the toublesome overhang.

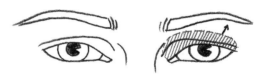

• *Droopy Eyes.* Yet another time-induced beauty problem! Gravity exerts its pull on all of us, and sooner or later your eyes can't help but take a downward turn at the outer corners. Counteract this by concentrating color and liner on the outer two-thirds of your lid. Join your upper and lower liner at the outer corner, and take both *very slightly* up and out beyond the natural outer corner. Curl your eyelashes upward, and be generous with mascara on your upper lashes.

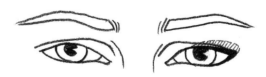

LUSTROUS NIGHTTIME LIPS

Let your lips dazzle at night! Rich, vibrant colors will balance out your stronger eye makeup. Opt for clear reds or russets. I particularly caution silver-haired women to avoid black-undertone colors, such as purple or cherry, which are hard and aging: Don't consider them even for Halloween! If you don't have a problem with lipstick bleeding into facial lines, finish off your evening lips with a slick of clear gloss. Apply it sparsely with your lip brush. Aim for luster—not gumminess.

7. Color Up

Color is critical to the way we look *and* the way we feel: exciting, confident, lively, glamorous, sexy. So I'm always sorry to see a woman take to wearing nothing but "safe" colors, such as blacks, grays, and browns, when her hair turns silver-gray. Many women do so because suddenly the colors that brought them to life when they were blondes or brunettes no longer seem quite right with their silver hair and lighter complexion.

The colors that suit you best don't actually change over the years. Because your genetics don't change, neither does your palette. *But you do need to rethink how you wear those colors.*

There's absolutely no reason to go into fashion mourning. Colors—whether in makeup or clothing—can brilliantly play up your best features and enhance your eyes, skin tone, and hair. Understanding color is essential to your look—learning to wield the proper palette can turn you from pale and drab to vibrant and glowing with youth. Here are some specific color principles for silver-haired women:

• Not all silver-haired women should use the same colors. "Having your colors done" has become an extremely popular notion in the past few years, and I think it has validity. I've seen a woman look like a million dollars in a simple T-shirt of the right color, but a silk designer gown in the *wrong* color can look cheap on her.

While every expert uses slightly different methods and labels, most agree that we all can be categorized as either cool or warm, depending on the pigmentation of our hair, skin, and eyes.

"Cool" denotes the side of the color wheel in which blue dominates. On it you'll find blue-reds, such as raspberry, fuchsia, and magenta, purple and violet, and blue-greens. If you are a cool person, your hair, skin, and eyes will have blue undertones, and you will have very little yellow pigmentation. (For the full story, see the color chart.) The hues on the cool side of the color wheel will suit you best. Elizabeth Taylor, with her raven hair, violet eyes, and alabaster skin is a typical cool beauty. But so is Linda Evans, with her ash-blond hair, gray-blue eyes, and soft pink skin.

Cool customers are lucky—their hair grays beautifully. Because of their lack of yellow pigmentation, once the brown and any red color they might have start to fade, their hair turns true silver.

"Warm" is represented by the side of the wheel in which yellow dominates: coral, tomato, orange, mustard, yellow-green. You will have

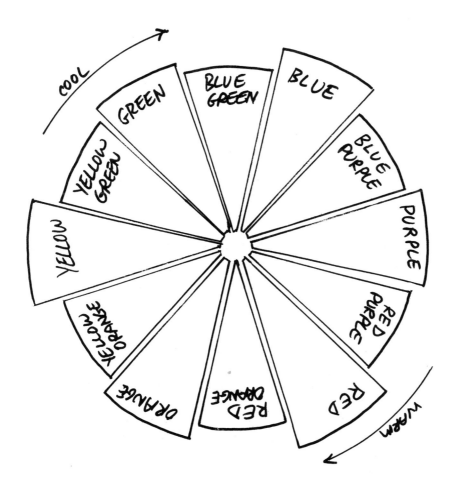

yellow pigmentation underlying your coloring, and look best in warm colors. A typical warm blonde is Catherine Deneuve, with her flaxen hair, green eyes, and creamy complexion. Victoria Principal—sherry-colored hair, velvety brown eyes, tan skin—embodies the darker end of the warm spectrum.

Warm-toned women are the ones who may need to give their silver hair an ashen rinse because it tends to have a yellowy cast. (Brown and red pigments fade first when your hair turns silver; the yellow is the last to go.) But don't make the mistake of thinking that when your hair turns silver, you automatically switch to the cool side of the wheel. Your skin tone and eyes are *still* warm and you should choose your colors accordingly.

Here's an easy-to-do at-home experiment to tell which side of the wheel you fall on, and what is your color identity:

Find two pieces of fabric—towels, sheets, or scarves are perfect—in the same general color (both red or both blue, for example), but make sure one is cool and the other is warm. Rose (representing cool) and peach (representing warm) are ideal. Now take off all your makeup and sit before a well-lit mirror. Hold up the cool color under your chin first, then the warm color.

You'll be astonished at the result. The "wrong" color very obviously will make your skin look washed-out and tired, show up any blemishes and wrinkles, make your eye color recede, and your hair dingy. But the "right" color will result in making your skin look radiant, your eyes intensified, and your hair shine. Try getting together with some friends to conduct this experiment. Then you can also compare skin tones, which makes it even easier to see the differences. I've recommended this test to many women, and they all have been surprised at how simple it is to figure out what classification they fall into.

In fact, you probably instinctively know what your best colors are. Think of your favorite item in your wardrobe. The one that you feel great in . . . that you wear on special occasions because it gives you confidence . . . your "lucky" outfit. Chances are, it is in a color from your correct palette. Now think of that lemon—the dress or blouse that looked so great in the pages of *Vogue* or in the window of Bloomingdale's, but never felt quite right on *you*. I'll guarantee it's the wrong color.

So what should you do if you have a closet full of lemons? No need to bundle them up for Goodwill just yet. Color-correct your wardrobe with the right-colored accessories until you gradually weed out all the wrong colors. Choose accessories from your own palette that complement the wrong-color garment. "Complementary" colors are those that lie across from each other on the color wheel, and they seem to bring out the best in each other. As you can see on the wheel, red complements green, blue complements orange, and so forth.

When possible, wear the right color near your face. For example, golden earrings and a yellow scarf tied at the throat will soften the effect of a navy sweater on a "warm" person who should never wear that shade of blue.

Here's a quick-reference chart listing your colors:

COOL

Original Hair Color:	Platinum, Nordic, or ash blond, light to dark brown, but always "mousy," blue-black.
Skin Tone:	Alabaster, milky, beige with rosy or pink-blue undertones, black with blue undertones. Pink cheeks. Cocoa-brown freckles.
Foundation:	Porcelain, fair, bisque, rose beige.
Cheek, Lip, Nail Colors:	Shell pink, peony, heather, watermelon, raspberry, plum, crimson, burgundy.
Eyes:	Blue-gray, light to slate gray, blue-green, taupe, and cocoa brown. Often have white flecks.
Eye Makeup:	Oyster, gunmetal, smoke, lilac, mulberry, wine, plum, navy, eggplant, hyacinth. Charcoal mascara.
Best Colors to Wear:	Bone, mushroom, all grays from silvery to charcoal; navy, royal, powder, denim blues; emerald and blue-greens; true and rose pink; blue-red, raspberry, burgundy, crimson, cardinal, and maroon; purple, violet, lilac, plum, and lavender; taupe; coffee and cocoa brown; soft black.
Worst Colors to Wear:	All golden browns; tan; mustard; yellow; peach; salmon; terra cotta; olive; khaki; jade; orange-reds, such as rust, brick, and tomato.
Jewelry:	Silver, white gold, platinum, rose pearls, diamonds, emeralds, aquamarines, opals, rose quartz, crystal, rhinestones.

WARM

Original Hair Color:	Flaxen, golden or strawberry blonde; chestnut or golden brown; auburn; carrot to copper red.
Skin Tone:	Ivory, peach, golden beige, black with copper undertones. Can be sallow or have peachy cheek color. Golden-brown freckles.
Foundation:	Cream, honey, ivory, rachel, sand, tan.
Cheek, Lip, Nail Colors:	Coral, apricot, ginger, russet, brick, rust, poppy, salmon, mocha, bronze, Indian earth.
Eyes:	Blue with gold flecks, pale or deep golden brown, hazel, amber.
Eye Makeup:	Earth tones, fawn, sepia, copper, pumpkin, brandy, olive, forest, ultramarine. Sable or brown-black mascara.
Best Colors to Wear:	Ivory, ecru, beige; golden and red browns—amber, ochre, bronze, fox, cinnamon; turquoise; yellows from saffron to daffodil; lime, olive, jade, and moss greens, khaki; peach, apricot, and salon pinks, clear and orange reds—brick, terra cotta, flame, Titian; brownish-black.
Worst Colors to Wear:	Gray, blue pinks and reds, navy, purple and burgundy, inky black, and pure white.
Jewelry:	Yellow gold, copper, brass, wood, ivory, amber, jade, turquoise, creamy pearls, topaz, and rubies.

• Now that you know what color palette suits you best, take a look at the *softer* end of the spectrum. Silver-haired women should opt for smoky, matted, and muted shades, rather than bright and glossy colors. I've never seen a silver-gray woman violate this rule and look good: Always avoid harshness in favor of softness. Crayon-brights and pop colors such as shocking pink, electric blue, chrome yellow, and acid green are just not going to work for you now.

Consider the degree to which your hair and complexion are lightening. The salt-and-pepper stage doesn't require the same muting that a mostly silver mane would dictate. The degree to which you mute your colors is always determined by the intensity of your personal "canvas"—hair, skin tone, and eyes. Remember that you're trying to complement your silver hair, not compensate for any reduction in natural color.

Use tones, shades, and tints rather than just pure colors, when designing your wardrobe. Pure colors are full-bodied, bold, brilliant, unadulterated: red, blue, yellow, green. But green is *not* always just green. With a dab of neutral white, gray, or black, or a splash of another primary color added, it can become mint, moss, jade, pea, bottle, lime, emerald, sage, forest, hunter, sea-foam, chartreuse, jungle, or olive! Think in terms of these *in-between* shades and you can't go far wrong.

• Use color to add some pizzazz to your life. One color from head to toe is dull, dull, dull! The monochromatic look is lacking in imagination, not to mention matronly. But don't go overboard. Four or more colors become strident. I think the ideal for clothing, as with eye makeup, is *three* colors—all, of course, from the correct side of the color wheel. For silver-haired women, the ideal combination is a *neutral*, plus a *basic* shade, plus a brighter *accent* color.

Either the neutral or the basic should dominate (about 70 percent to 20 percent), while your accent adds just a touch (about 10 percent) of the total color.

Generally, the dominant color is your dress, suit, skirt, or pants. The secondary color is for blouses, T-shirts, jackets, sweaters, stockings, and sometimes accessories. And your accent color is for belts, scarves, jewelry, bags, shoes, hats, or anywhere you want to draw attention to.

Again, with your silver hair, you should stick to *low-contrast* combinations—muted shades—rather than clashing or garish colors. For example, tone pale neutrals with medium basic shades, medium neutrals with dark basic shades, and dark neutrals with medium basic shades. Your accent color should have the same intensity as the darker of the two colors. The exception (isn't there always one?) is those combinations—black and white; red, white, and blue—that are such classics, they defy the rules.

Some dynamic three-way combinations for cool-toned women: pearl gray, dusty pink, and purple . . . white, navy, and raspberry . . . black, steel gray, and violet . . . bone, mushroom, and taupe . . . white, washed-out denim blue, and crimson . . . mushroom, black, and royal blue . . . cool beige, deep rose, and emerald.

And great three-way combinations for warm-toned women: ecru, olive green, and mustard . . . ivory, walnut brown, and teal blue . . . sand, russet, and tomato . . . cream, peach, and turquoise . . . pale yellow, orange, and lime green . . . warm beige, coral, and forest green.

A Word About White

Scientists have found that the human eye automatically goes to lightest hues first and then, in descending order, to the darker colors. It happens in a flash; nevertheless, the impression is made. This is good news for silver-haired women, since it means that your luminous hair makes an *instant impact*.

Bear this principle in mind, however, when choosing your wardrobe. White and other pale, light-reflecting tones will draw attention, emphasize, and give the illusion of weight, darker shades tend to minimize. Take care then to use white only where and when you want to be noticed.

A Word About Black

Black is the eternally chic color: It's classic, sophisticated, worldly and powerful. Not for nothing has the "little black dress" been the staple of many a P.M. wardrobe for decades and decades.

Black is truly an adult color, and you have the panache now to carry it off as never before. *But* your silver hair does place some limitations on you.

The contrast between a black outfit and your light hair can look harsh. Cool women can wear it more effectively than warm, because true black is a cool color. Evaluate yourself very carefully in all lights before opting to wear black. Does it cast shadows on your face? Drain color from your cheeks? Emphasize lines? Make you look tired? If so:

• Avoid jet or inky black in favor of softer versions of "off"-black colors, such as charcoal, grayed navy, blackish burgundy (for cool women) . . . bitter chocolate and deep forest green (for warm).

• Choose "soft" fabrics, such as velvet or satin, that reflect light as you move. Also consider beaded or sequined outfits—they have the same effect. Wear black lace *over* a brighter-colored lining.

• Wear a black dress or suit but soften it with a brighter, softer color in a blouse, scarf, or wrap near your face.

PART IV

THE TOTAL PICTURE

8. Body Work

There's a reason why massages, herbal wraps, manicures, and pedicures are priorities for La Costa guests. Face and hair may express your style more than anything, but smart women know it doesn't end there. Your body, smile, and hands are part of the total picture. Glamour is a top-to-toe proposition, but it doesn't have to be an all-day affair. Here's a scan down your body and a program for keeping your total appeal at a maximum in the minimum possible time.

TIPS FOR HEALTHY, DAZZLING TEETH

There's nothing like a drop-dead smile. Good news! You don't have to accept tooth decay or a receding gum line as an immutable fact. Such tremendous strides have occurred in orthodontics and periodontics in recent years that your teeth can be beautiful and healthy forever. In fact, you're much less prone to cavities now than when you were a teenager, although you need to pay close attention to your gums: The incidence of periodontal disease (and the danger of losing your teeth) increases sharply in later life. Begin to take maintenance care right *now*, and you'll have a better-than-excellent chance of having healthy teeth and a dazzling smile your entire life.

The first and most important step is to combat plaque—the thin film that coats your teeth and interacts with bacteria. If you don't remove it, it hardens into tartar, which causes gum disease. That in turn leads to a receding line and possible tooth loss. To eliminate plaque, you must see your dentist every four months for a checkup and a professional cleaning and follow this simple daily routine. It's the most up-to-date thinking on what works.

• Brush your teeth after breakfast, using a fluoride toothpaste and a medium/soft toothbrush with round-ended bristles. Replace your toothbrush about every three months or when the bristles have become splayed. The American Dental Association recommends aligning bristles with the gum line at a forty-five degree angle and brushing with a short, gentle, scrubbing motion.

• Brush again after lunch or snacking during the day. Impractical? At least rinse your mouth with water, especially after eating sweet or sticky foods.

• Before you go to bed, make a paste of baking soda and peroxide (which you can buy at your drugstore) and brush your teeth thoroughly with the paste for several minutes. Floss between your teeth with waxed dental floss (Johnson & Johnson makes both a mint- and a cinnamon-flavored kind to make the job more palatable), and use a Water Pik appliance. Give your teeth a final brushing with toothpaste if you like the fresh taste in your mouth.

Using a baking-soda-and-peroxide mix is fairly controversial among dentists. Many feel that it isn't *what* you brush with; it's the brushing itself that does the cleaning. The peroxide, however, does help with another problem—discolored teeth. Coffee drinking, eating, smoking: They're all culprits in staining teeth. The thinning of tooth enamel over the years can also make your teeth appear darker.

If you are faced with this discoloration, avoid wearing orange, bronze, or brown lipstick—these colors only emphasize the staining. Pink and blue/pink shades, on the other hand, make your teeth appear whiter.

Enamel bonding is a *permanent* solution to the problem of stained teeth. An ultrathin veneer of porcelain or plastic is painted on your teeth to color-correct or fill in problem areas. The material literally "bonds" with the tooth enamel itself (unlike a bridge or a crown, which is *attached* to the problem tooth). Bonding will cover stains, mend chips, even out worndown teeth, and close gaps by becoming part of the actual tooth. The technique has become widely available over the last couple of years, and is much less expensive than bridges or crowns. I've seen some fabulous results among my clients from bonding.

Loss of teeth despite your best efforts, however, no longer necessarily means dentures. Implanting or transplanting individual teeth is now a possibility. This method results in a look that's more natural than full or partial plates. Ask your dentist if you are a suitable candidate for the procedure: In some cases, gum disease makes it impossible.

KEEPING YOUR BODY TRIM AND FIT

I don't know a single person who is completely happy with her body. Instead of looking at ourselves kindly—all those years of dedicated service!—we focus on the flaws. It's crucial to your physical and emotional well-being for you to *love* your body. One way to go about getting to that state is to discover (if you haven't already) the pleasure of exercise.

The way to go about it? If you haven't exercised much to date, get a complete physical and your doctor's go-ahead to start a program. Set realistic goals, find activities you thoroughly *enjoy* (it's the only way you'll stick with it), and get support and encouragement by joining a club or group of like-minded people.

The ideal combination is an aerobic activity (swimming, walking, running, dancing, cycling) for fat-burning and cardiovascular health; stretching (stretch classes or yoga) for grace and flexibility; strength work (calisthenics or light weights) for body sculpting. It's the closest humankind has come to an antiaging pill! You'll be vigorous and alert, and your skin tone will be clear, your energy level sky-high. Plus, of course, you'll be trim and fit. A stable weight through sound diet and exercise is the linchpin for overall beauty.

CARING FOR YOUR BODY SKIN

Your face has certainly borne the brunt of attack from the elements—sun, wind, and pollution—but the rest of your body skin also tends to dry with time. Treat particularly rough or callused areas—elbows and heels—by rubbing lightly with a pumice stone and moisturizing, and get into the habit of total body-skin care. It entails the same general principles as facial care: cleanse, exfoliate, moisturize.

• *Cleanse.* When your skin tends toward dryness, stick to showering in warm water rather than soaking in a hot bath. Even bath oil won't prevent the water from leaching moisture out of your skin, leaving it dry, scaly, and sometimes itchy. If you shower more than once a day because you exercise or have a job that gets you dirty, be particularly conscientious about skin care—take brief showers in tepid-to-cool water.

Use a mild soap with a high fat content, such as Dove. *Never* use deodorant brands, which have too many potentially irritating additives. It's my belief that the whole "squeaky-clean" mythology is overdone. We're much too fanatical about odor masking. If you wash daily and use an antiperspirant after showering, you'll be perfecty fine. If you like, dust

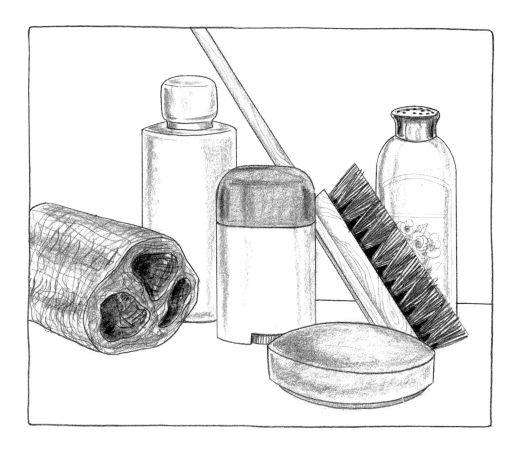

with scented talc or baby powder to keep feeling fresh. (Confine powder to your upper body. Do not dust between your legs, around your genital area, or inside your panties, as talc has been linked to cervical cancer.)

• *Exfoliate.* Your body collects debris and dead skin cells, just as your face does. Slough them off regularly to keep your skin clear and soft. You can use your facial exfoliant—although you may find that extravagant. My personal favorite overall exfoliant is a loofah—a natural, vegetable sponge, available in most drugstores for a couple of dollars. Wet the loofah, soap it up, and *gently* rub your whole body in a circular motion. Our loofah rub is one of La Costa's most popular pampering extras. A soft-bristle body brush or a mitt of rough fabric used in the same way will also do the job. Don't scrub hard; you don't need to see red in order to see results.

Exfoliate your body once a week. Pay special attention to rough spots, such as elbows, knees, and feet. Your body will tingle from the increased circulation, and your skin will feel like silk—I guarantee it!

• *Moisturize.* When you step out of the shower, pat your body with a fluffy cotton towel, and while you're still damp, slather on a body lotion. Most body lotions have a lower oil content than the moisturizer you use on your face, and "disappear" on your skin fairly quickly. In hot, dry, or cold and windy weather, reapply it to your arms and legs during the day.

PAMPER YOUR HANDS

After the eyes, I think a woman's hands are the most expressive part of her persona. Don't neglect something so vital and visible! After all, the skin on your hands is subject to the same aging processes as facial skin: It becomes dry and flaky, it wrinkles, it thins and shows veins, and it develops brown spots. Some of these conditions are made worse by wear and tear, but *all* of them can be helped!

• *Always* wear rubber gloves when working in water. Forget those commercials for dishwashing liquid that promise soft, silky hands! Plunging them into hot, dirty water several times a day means, rough, scaly skin and brittle nails. Keep a pair of sturdy gloves by the sink, and don't even turn on the faucet until you have slipped them on.

• Stand a bottle of hand lotion by every sink or washbasin in your home, and use it—religiously! For an extra treat, smooth hand lotion on *before* you put on your gloves. The heat from the water will give you a beauty treatment while you're working.

• Carry a small tube or bottle of hand cream in your purse, and don't wait until your hands feel dry before applying it. Moisturize after you wash or wet your hands, while they are still slightly damp (to seal in the water). Use a cream *with sunscreen* especially formulated for hands. It will have a heavier oil content and cling to your skin more than lotions made for your face or body.

• Make it a point to wear gloves when you are working with harsh detergents, chemical substances, or in the garden. Gardening with gloves protects your hands from dirt and scrapes while providing a barrier against the sun.

Remember: The sun is usually the cause of brown spots on the backs of your hands. You cannot have them removed by cosmetic surgery or cover them with makeup, as you can when they appear on your face, and "fade" creams are only partially effective. So *prevention* is worth the trouble. Supplement the sunscreen in your hand lotion with a strong sun block when you are spending any time out of doors.

• In winter, protect your hands from cold, wind, and rain by wearing gloves at all times when you are out. Fingernails also take a beating in winter. Both the cold outside and overheated rooms sap the natural moisture from your nails. While we're on the subject, let's talk about nails some more.

A REGULAR NAIL-CARE ROUTINE

Fingernails tend to be the focal point of your hands. They grow a little more slowly and become more brittle with each passing decade, so a regular nail-care routine is essential.

Nails, like hair, are almost pure dead protein—the only part of your nail that is growing is the *fold*, which starts at the cuticle and extends under the skin for a couple of millimeters. An injury to that part of your finger—such as trapping it in a drawer—will show up as a black bruise or white spots, and because your nails grow about one-sixteenth of an inch per week, you'll be stuck with the deformity for several months.

Other unusual discolorations, ridges, pits, and splitting may indicate bad nutrition or ill health. Your nails (like your hair) are particularly susceptible to dysfunctions of your thyroid gland. An overactive gland tends to cause the nail to pull away from your finger; an underactive gland results in dry, breakable nails.

If you have nails that break easily, there is a temptation to wear full or partial false nails made from porcelain or acrylics. But in all cases, the

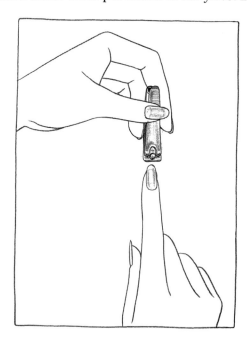

techniques and glues used can weaken your nails even further. Once you start wearing them, it's hard to stop, because your own nails underneath are such a mess. I'm generally not in favor of such procedures.

The following seven-step weekly manicure will keep your *own* nails in great shape:

• Take off your polish with a cotton ball soaked with remover. Polish remover can be drying, so get one that comes in an oil base—such as Cutex Oily Polish Remover—and do not use it more than once a week.

• Trim your nails straight across with a nail clipper. Long, clawlike nails are unfashionable and unflattering, not to mention impractical, for most women. One-quarter of an inch beyond the fingertip is currently the style and is as long as anyone should wear her nails.

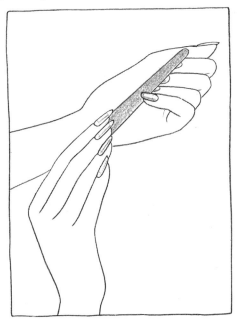

• With an emery board, smooth nails into a square-off oval. Nails look pretty when the shape of the tip mirrors the curve of the base. This contour will give your nails the most strength. Filing them to a point will weaken them and make them prone to splitting.

• Soak your fingertips for about a minute in warm water to which a drop of bath or baby oil has been added. If your nails are particularly brittle, soak them in warmed baby oil. Nails are very absorbent, and the oil will make them more pliant. Pat your hands dry and massage in a rich hand cream, taking care to include your cuticle area.

• Using an orange stick wrapped with cotton, gently push back your cuticles. Clip any hangnails from the sides of your cuticles.

• Wipe polish remover over your nails to take off any oily residue before you paint them.

• If you want to underplay your hands and nails, go for the unvarnished truth by simply buffing your nails to a natural shine with a chamois-covered nail buffer.

Be bolder if you wish to draw attention to pretty hands. Apply a coat of clear base coat. While it is still tacky, apply a couple of coats of nail color, and finish with a slick of clear top coat extended over the ends to the undersides of your nails. The procedure: Start with pinkies and work in to thumbs. Paint your right hand first *if* you're right-handed, and vice versa (you're most adroit with your "good" hand, so are less likely to smudge fresh color when painting the second hand). Apply polish in three brush strokes—one down the middle and one on each side. Clean up mistakes with a cotton swab dipped in remover.

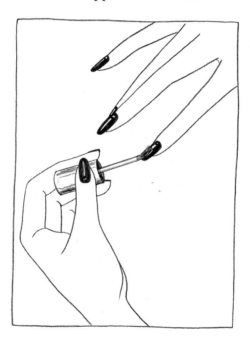

As for colors, choose translucent glazes or mid-range creme enamels, such as rose, coral, peach, and ginger for daytime wear. Be more adventurous at night, and branch out with bright, zingy reds, wines, and frosted polishes. Avoid chalky pastels and purples with black undertones.

When you don't have time to sit and let polish dry, use one of the "fast-drying" products. I like Revlon's Non-Dulling Quick Dry aerosol spray. You can get a similar effect by dipping your nails in ice-cold water. Remember, both techniques only dry the top layer; you still need to take care for half an hour to let undercoats dry.

FOR PRETTY FEET

"My feet are killing me!" How many times have you said that? Feet can indeed be a dead giveaway of age. Think of all the damage you've inflicted on them over the years! Luckily, most of that can be remedied, and with care and attention, your feet can be comfortable, pretty . . . even sexy!

The biggest cause of unattractive feet is ill-fitting shoes. Take time and care when buying shoes to make sure that they do not rub or bind your heel or big-toe joint. There should also be plenty of room in the toe. Pad around the house barefoot at every opportunity, to give your feet a break from being squeezed.

Be scrupulous about foot hygiene—we often forget to soap our feet in the shower. Wash, rinse, and dry them well, especially between your toes, in order to prevent redness, itching, or a breeding place for fungus. Dust your feet with baby powder or special foot powder before slipping into your stockings and shoes. Once a week, treat yourself to a home pedicure:

• Soak your feet for ten minutes in a bowl of warm water mixed with half a cup of Epsom salts and a few drops of bath oil. You'll feel wonderfully relaxed, in addition to softening your skin and nails.

• With a soft-bristled nail brush, scrub your toenails to remove any dirt from underneath.

• Dip a pumice stone in the water, and then gently rub away any callused or hard skin. Pay particular attention to your heels. If you

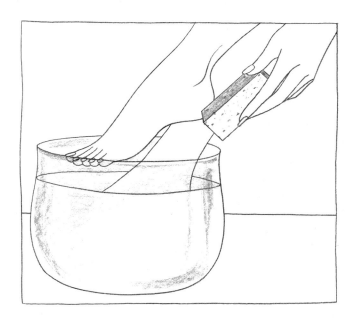

regularly wear high heels, you probably also have a wad of compacted skin on the ball of your foot. Do not rub too vigorously. You will not be able to remove all the dead skin at one time, but if you use the pumice stone regularly, the layers will eventually wear down.

• Rinse your feet and dry them thoroughly, especially between the toes.

• Clip your toenails *straight across*, not rounded off, like fingernails, and not so short that they do not protect the ends of your toes. Use an emery board to smooth rough edges that might catch on your hose.

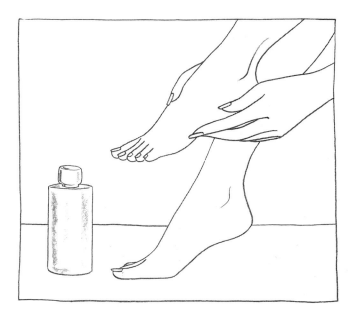

• Pour a rich hand or body lotion on to your feet and massage it in, starting at the ball of each foot. Work the lotion around your toes, all along the soles and heels. Knead well with your fingertips—really massage out the kinks and sore spots!

• While the lotion is still on your feet, use an orange stick wrapped with cotton to push back the cuticles on your toenails. Be gentle!

• Wipe the lotion off your toenails with a cotton ball soaked in nail-polish remover. (Otherwise, the oily lotion will prevent nail polish from adhering.)

• Want to show off your pretty feet in sandals? Paint your toenails with one layer of base coat, a couple of coats of polish the same shade as your fingernails, and a top coat. A professional tip for making toenail painting easier: Twist a tissue into a cylinder and weave it between your toes to separate them before painting.

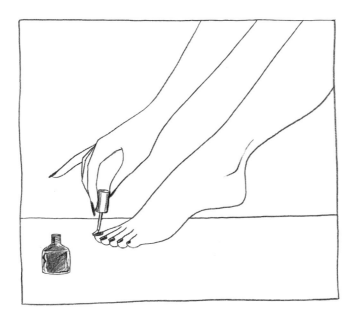

If you don't want to draw attention to your feet, forget about the color. Just buff your nails to a natural shine and give them a slick of clear polish.

• Maintain your nails through the week by touching up any chipped color.

I recommend an occasional professional pedicure. Nothing makes you feel more pampered than having someone massage your feet! Furthermore, your pedicurist might spot developing problems that require a visit to the podiatrist. Be on the alert for the most common of these ailments.

• *Athlete's foot* is a fungal infection. You will know you have it if you itch between your toes—where it usually starts—and notice redness, tiny blisters, and scaly skin. Try an over-the-counter remedy, and see your doctor if there's no improvement.

• *Blisters* are caused by friction from too-tight or new shoes. Avoid the troublemakers until the blisters are healed. In the meantime, do not be tempted to burst the blisters—that might lead to an infection. Should they pop of their own accord, wash the area and cover with a Band-Aid.

• *Bunions* are a painful and unsightly deformity of the big toe joint. Wear shoes big enough to accommodate them—shoes that are too tight will result in the area's becoming even more red and swollen. Bunions should always be looked at by a doctor, since they could be an indication of arthritis.

• *Corns*—layers of compacted skin formed as protection when shoes rub on bony areas—are one of the most common foot problems. Remove them gradually by rubbing regularly with a pumice stone or foot file. *Never* try to cut them away, since broken skin can lead to infection.

• *Ingrown toenails* can be prevented by clipping your nails straight across, not curved at the sides. If you do get nails that are painfully imbedded in your skin, minor surgery might be required to repair the situation.

• *Unpleasant foot odor* can be embarrassing. Actually, it's probably your shoes and stockings—not your feet—that are the culprits, even though your feet have thousands of sweat glands that exude about half a pint of perspiration in an average day. Your shoes absorb the sweat, which becomes contaminated by bacteria that begin to give off an odor. Thorough washing (with Betadine solution in severe cases) helps combat a chronic problem.

Wear clean socks or stockings every day, and alternate pairs of shoes so that each pair has a chance to air out. Natural materials breathe better than man-made, so if odor is a problem, opt for cotton or wool socks, silk stockings, and leather shoes.

FRAGRANT FACTS

Nothing is more womanly, more personal, more evocative— and elicits more emotional response—than the scent you wear. Millions of women may spray on your fragrance . . . but the moment it touches *your* skin it becomes undeniably your own. Body chemistry, interacting with the oils and extracts in the perfume, makes scent a surprisingly *unique* statement.

I know that perfume is considered a perfect gift, but I think that unless you know a person's preferred fragrance, a gift of perfume is a mistake. In the bottle and on the skin are two different stories. Don't pay a substantial amount of money for a new fragrance until you (or your planned recipient) have tested it. After all, that's why perfume counters always have testers.

Test a perfume by spraying or dabbing a little on your wrist. Then walk away, and come back the next day! You won't get the full effect of how a perfume reacts to your chemistry for several hours. Perfumes usually have three "notes." The top note is what you detect immediately after you have applied the scent

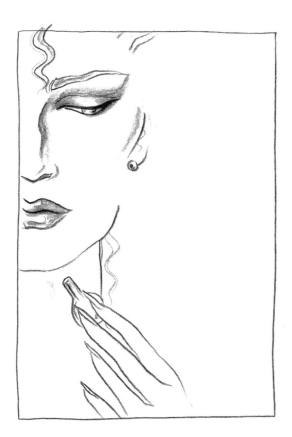

(it tends to fade in about fifteen minutes). Then you notice the middle note (which lasts about half an hour). Finally, the base note emerges. This is the true essence, which takes awhile to develop but lingers for several hours. Only when the scent has completed this cycle can you truly tell if a particular perfume is right for you.

I find scents difficult to describe in words, because they're a totally *sensual* experience. Even so, they generally can be characterized as floral, spicy, musky, woodsy, or Oriental, according to the predominant flowers or essences they contain. You might not be able to place a particular scent, but chances are that all your personal favorites belong to the same category!

There are two schools of thought on perfume. Some people believe you should establish a "signature" scent—one that becomes emphatically associated with you. Then there are those who favor capriciousness—wearing whatever strikes your mood at a given time. The choice is completely yours: This is an area where there are no rules; there's only the delight of indulging in whatever takes your fancy.

Scent comes in various forms. In descending order of strength and durability, there is perfume or *parfum, parfum de toilette, eau de toilette,* and cologne. Don't buy the largest-size bottle of perfume—it's prone to evaporation and spoiling. Keep your scents in a cool, dark place to give them the best chance of staying fresh until you've used them up. For a more subtle effect than perfume, use soaps, talcs, bath oils, and body lotions in your favorite scent.

Finally, be artful with your perfume. Your scent should never precede you into a room or linger after you have gone. The idea is to give off an almost elusive fragrance that draws people a little closer to you.

9. Buying Beauty

osmetic surgery has become the fastest-growing medical specialty in the nation. What was once the preserve of the rich and famous is now within reach of almost anyone who wants to take advantage of improved techniques and more affordable prices. And why not? Wanting to look your best, whether it's to feel better about yourself or to compete in the work force, is no longer considered vanity. *There's nothing wrong with wanting to look as young as you feel.*

Questions about *cosmetic* (or aesthetic) surgery—as opposed to *reconstructive* plastic surgery—rank at the top of the list for the women who visit our spa. I think it's such an important and sometimes confusing issue that I've compiled a roundup of the major services available to give you an idea of what's happening in this fast-changing field.

Before I do that, however, I *can* advise you, based on countless conversations I've had with women, that if you think a face-lift or eye tuck is going to cure some deeper-seated unhappiness, you'll be severely disappointed. A correction here or there will not save a failing marriage or win you a promotion. *Rejuvenating surgery is for enhancement, not magical results.*

Don't underestimate the seriousness of any surgery. Many of these procedures can cause temporary swelling, bruising, bleeding, scarring, and discomfort. Also, they often require considerable recovery time. Because everyone heals differently, results cannot be guaranteed with any of these treatments. You must be highly motivated not only to invest a certain amount of money and time, but to undergo discomfort as well.

HOW TO CHOOSE A PLASTIC SURGEON

Esthetic surgery is usually sought for cosmetic purposes—not because you're ill—but don't forget that it is nonetheless *surgery,* and as such has the same attendant risks as any other operation. Take it from someone who's seen many and varied results on clients. *Choose your surgeon very carefully.*

Any physician can legally hang out a shingle that says "Cosmetic Surgeon," but that does not necessarily mean that he or she is certified by the American Board of Plastic Surgery. In order to get that certification, the doctor must have had at least three years' training in plastic surgery and have passed rigorous written and oral examinations. *Never be shy about asking your doctor if he or she is board certified, and don't even consider undergoing plastic surgery with anyone who is not.* So how do you find a suitable qualified doctor?

In 1979, the Federal government ruled that doctors could advertise their services. The medical profession is still split on this decision. Those against it claim that doctors who spend thousands of dollars in advertising use the "conveyor belt" approach with patients, and that people are not given enough individual attention.

Those in favor think that they are bringing information about these erstwhile exclusive procedures to "Everyman." By treating a high volume of patients, they can keep costs down, making it affordable to most who want to undergo plastic surgery.

Selecting a plastic surgeon calls for careful consideration. I think you're much better off finding a surgeon by referral than through an advertisement (*walking* evidence of someone's skills, not just a written come-hither). Ask friends for recommendations. Also be sure to consult your primary-care physician, and you can call your local hospital for the names of some suitable candidates. Failing that, get in touch with The American Society of Plastic and Reconstructive Surgery, 233 North Michigan Avenue, Chicago, Illinois 60601. The Society will provide you with a list of surgeons in your area, and will also answer any questions you have about a doctor's qualifications.

Once you have some names, arrange a consultation with two or three doctors. (You've come this far; *don't* close your eyes and barrel ahead with the first likely choice!) I recommend checking for the following:

- The doctor should allow you sufficient time to ask all your questions about the procedure, and should answer you frankly and fully.
- The doctor should inquire into your reasons—both physical and psychological—for wanting the surgery. *Never* let yourself be pushed into something you don't want to do.
- Ask the doctor to show you some photographs of his or her work, including before-and-after shots. Your interest will be *appreciated.*
- Get a detailed description of the operation, the recovery time, and the possible risks, complications, and side effects. Does the doctor tell you honestly what scars will result and what are the maximum effects you can achieve?
- Is the doctor prepared to give you a detailed and firm quote on the cost of treatment?
- Check to make sure that the doctor's facility is fully equipped with life support systems, should an emergency arise during the operation. Does he or she have a suitably qualified person administering the anesthetic?
- Do you feel a rapport with the doctor . . . comfortable about the prospect of literally putting your face in his or her hands? *I urge you never to underestimate the importance of feeling at ease with your surgeon's professional skills* and *personal demeanor.*

A number of procedures are available, from the relatively simple, which can be done in a doctor's office, to major surgery, requiring hospitalization. In the following catalog, I've skipped such restructuring operations as "nose jobs" or breast augmentation, in order to concentrate on rejuvenation therapies.

REPLACEMENT THERAPY

Certain facial lines are plumped up by injections of a filler material in this nonsurgical technique. Years ago, doctors used liquid silicone, but this artificial substance was found to migrate to other parts of the body, and is no longer sanctioned by the Federal Drug Administration (FDA) for this purpose. (Injectable silicone is different from the silicone implants used in breast augmentation or cheek and chin implants.)

Since 1981 Zyderm® Collagen has been the most common replacement for liquid silicone. It is a purified animal substance similar to your body's own collagen, and bonds with it to smooth out wrinkles. Most effective treatment areas? Frown lines, vertical lines around your mouth, and nasal-labia folds—the creases that run from your nose to your mouth. It cannot fix crow's feet around your eyes, or the fine lines that network your cheeks.

You must be tested before a collagen treatment to make sure you are not allergic to it. Your dermatologist or cosmetic surgeon will inject a little into your forearm, and will check the site in seventy-two hours and then again in a month, to see if there is a reaction. According to Dr. Peter Goldman, a Los Angeles dermatologist, who was one of pioneering researchers involved in the procedure, about 97 percent of those tested have no adverse reaction. A small number (0.5 percent) of those who show no allergy during the test, later have a reaction on their faces . . . so your odds of being a suitable candidate are quite high.

The procedure involves injecting small drops of the liquid—which comprises 30 percent collagen, 70 percent water, and a minute amount of pain-killer—directly into the line. You might need between two and six treatments before a wrinkle is filled in—it can be awfully persistent! Expect some swelling and bruising for a day or two, but when it subsides—smooth, clear skin.

To date, the only drawback of collagen has been that it breaks down, over time, the way your own collagen did originally. You need to have touch-up shots—although in smaller amounts—once or twice a year. However, scientists are working to produce a more permanent collagen. In fact, a new version, called Glutaraldehyde Cross-Linked Collagen (GAX), has just been introduced on the market, and appears to have longer-lasting effects.

Another variation on this replacement-therapy theme is to use fibroplast instead of collagen. It's derived from your own blood—no allergic reaction! A vial of blood is drawn from your arm in the doctor's office, processed on the spot into a protein substance similar to collagen, and injected right into the wrinkle. Thereafter, it's much like collagen—*except* that there's an even greater "fade factor." Plan on fairly frequent booster shots.

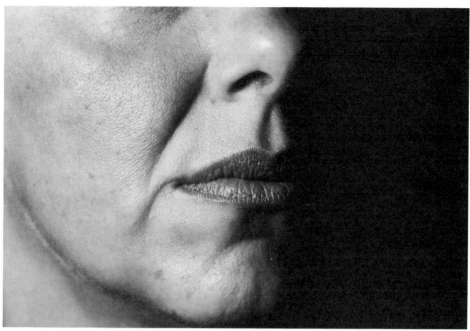

Aging lines before Zyderm® collagen treatments (COURTESY COLLAGEN CORPORATION)

Aging lines after Zyderm® collagen treatments (COURTESY COLLAGEN CORPORATION)

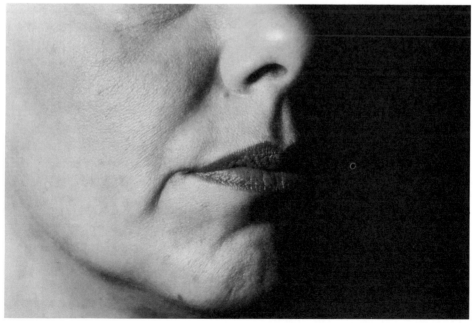

RESURFACING THERAPY

This technique involves removing the top layer of your skin to allow fresh, new growth to form. It helps eliminate the fine lines that neither implants nor face-lifts will eradicate. The procedure can be performed at any age, either when these lines first appear, or in later life in conjunction with a face-lift.

The best results are achieved on fair-skinned women with light eyes. Resurfacing can leave uneven patches of pigmentation and cause scarring on blacks, Orientals, and oily-skinned, swarthy Caucasians. But Nature has a way of balancing these things out, because light-skinned women are the ones most prone to the type of premature wrinkling on which resurfacing works best.

Resurfacing on *small* patches of skin can be accomplished through *cryosurgery*, which involves the use of liquid nitrogen to freeze blemishes such as brown spots. But the two common techniques that can be used on much larger areas, or even on the entire face, are dermabrasion and chemical peeling.

These resurfacing therapies are booming, but please don't take them lightly. You're dealing with very strong chemicals, not to mention a relatively long recovery period and increased vulnerability to the sun. Make sure you're a perfect candidate for these procedures before you say, "yes"!

Dermabrasion

Dermabrasion—or "sanding"—is a mechanical method most often used to smooth out acne pits, pockmarks, and scars, although it's also good for removing freckles, brown spots, fine wrinkles, and other superficial skin irregularities. You can have either specific areas or your entire face sanded. Usually only one session is necessary, but if more sessions are needed, they can be done about three months apart.

The process itself is painless, takes about two hours, and is performed in the dermatologist's or plastic surgeon's office while you are under local anesthetic. The doctor uses a fast-rotating steel wire brush or diamond-studded disc to sand the surface of your face, much as a carpenter would plane a plank of wood.

Within a couple of days, a tight protective crust forms, which can cause intense throbbing. Your doctor will give you pain-relievers for this. Later, as your face heals under the scab, it may begin to itch. Resist—at all costs—the mighty temptation to scratch or pick at the crust—it could result in scarring. During the recovery time, you might have to stick to a liquid diet, because you will not be able to move your mouth to chew. Also, you will not be able to wash your hair during this period.

Within ten to fourteen days, the crust will fall away, revealing the newly formed skin underneath. This smooth, fresh skin will be pink for a couple of months, here's where makeup comes to the rescue. About two weeks after receiving treatment, you can easily camouflage it and resume your normal life.

You *must*—no exceptions—protect your face from the sun for at least six weeks, and preferably six months, after dermabrasion. It is the most important point I can make about insuring good results. If you're deliberately cavalier, you run the risk of developing a condition called hyperpigmentation, which is blotchy brown patches.

Chemical Peeling

Chemical peeling, also known as chemosurgery, has the same results as dermabrasion, but the method is quite different. In this case, a caustic agent is painted onto your face that literally eats away the top layers of skin.

The mildest form of peel involves the use of trichloroacetic acid (TCA). The solution is applied without anesthetic in the doctor's office once a week for several weeks. It burns slightly on application for a few minutes. Your face will feel tight for a couple of days, and then the top layer of skin will shed, just like a snake's. After a couple of sessions, you will be down to fresh skin—minus the superficial wrinkles and discolorations.

More commonly, though, chemical peeling is done in one session, with a much stronger acid, called phenol. It takes off several layers of skin, almost as though you have received a controlled second-degree burn. Obviously, this more severe technique carries the risk of more side effects.

Your doctor should insist that you have a complete physical before you undergo chemosurgery. This is because minute amounts of the toxic chemical are absorbed by the skin, enter the bloodstream, and can cause problems in anyone with kidney, liver, or heart irregularities.

The procedure can be performed in the doctor's office, although it's often done in a hospital. Expect a tingling or stinging sensation for up to an hour after the solution is painted onto your face. Shortly after that, your face will begin to swell—and the swelling will last for several hours and can feel quite painful. Don't be alarmed by what looks like discoloration at this point, it's normal and temporary.

If you are having a light peel, you will be sent home to wait for the dead skin to flake off. *Under no circumstances should you pull at the skin as it begins to curl away from your face.* You can, however, very carefully snip off the dead tissue with clean nail scissors. As with dermabrasion, you must also resist scratching the healing skin.

If your doctor has decided that you need a heavier peel, he or she will apply a tape to your face on top of the chemical, which allows the solution to work on deeper layers of your skin. The tape mask is left on for one or two days, during which you should remain fairly still and will not be able to talk much or eat solid food. But at least you'll be encouraged to take hot baths and drink hot liquids to promote sweating and increase the flow of serum to your skin.

When the tape is removed, the doctor will shake an antiseptic powder onto your face. You'll get your own supply to use as often as necessary until a dry, firm crust forms. Thereafter the story is the same as with dermabrasion: initial tightness and throbbing, scab falls off in about two weeks, face pink for a couple of months, sun *must* be avoided.

There is one possible permanent effect of chemosurgery. The peeled area might end up paler than the unpeeled areas, leaving a demarcation line around your chin, because some skin pigmentation will have been removed from the epidermal layers. The only solution at this point, unfortunately, is to camouflage the problem with makeup. You cannot peel your neck or any other part of your body to match, because severe scarring could occur.

SURGICAL TECHNIQUES FOR FACIAL REPAIRS

So much for handling the superficial appearance of your skin. What about the problems of sagging muscles and fatty deposits? Those require "aesthetic" surgery—the surgeon actually goes under the skin and alters the underlying structure of your face.

Blepharoplasty

Blepharoplasty, or eyelid surgery, is one of the most commonly performed reconstructive operations. According to the American Society of Plastic and Reconstructive Surgeons, only breast augmentation is more asked-for. Eyelid surgery effectively eliminates heavy, droopy upper lids and undereye pouches.

Some people are genetically programmed to have these characteristics from childhood. But even if you are not, you might develop them later in life. As your skin and muscles lose their elasticity, fatty deposits push through this flagging support system. In extreme cases, your eyelids can droop so much that they begin to obscure your vision.

You can safely have this condition corrected at any age, from teens to seventies. Because it is performed strictly on the external part of the eye, diseases such as glaucoma or cataracts need not deter you. (But don't forget to inform your surgeon about the condition and any medication you are taking for it.)

The operation should be performed in a hospital or clinic that has good pre- and post-operative facilities. It takes a couple of hours, and you are usually given a local anesthetic, so that you can move your eyes during the procedure. Most doctors also put you on an intravenous tranquilizer.

Incisions are made in the fold of your upper lid and along the lash line on the lower lid. Excess fat and overstretched muscles are removed. The cuts are sutured with very fine material. You should stay in bed for the first day after the procedure and take it easy for the next week—be sure not to do any exercise or stooping. Also, wear sunglasses to protect your eyes from the elements and to help you remember not to rub your eyes inadvertently.

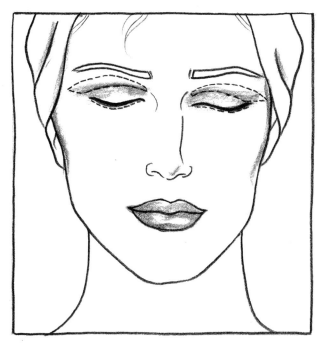

The cuts made in eyelid surgery are invisible, as they are made in the fold of your lids.

You might have some bruising and swelling for a couple of days. Don't be alarmed if your vision is a little blurred at first; it's only because of the swelling. You will be back to normal as soon as the puffiness subsides. In most cases, you can start wearing eye makeup within a week and resume all usual activity within ten days. If you wear contacts, you might have to wait another week, because the usual manhandling of your lids is still too much for them at this early post-operative stage.

Any more lasting reminders? Just some fine scars that will fade with time, but not to worry—they'll be practically invisible in the meantime, because they are located in the natural creases of your eyes.

Rhytidectomy

Rhytidectomy is the clinical name for a face-lift. The function of a lift is to reverse the downcast look that results from the tug of gravity on your jowls, brows, cheeks, and mouth, and to firm up skin that has lost some of its elasticity and is now sagging.

The effects of a lift can last anywhere from two to fifteen years, depending on the state of the skin when the operation was performed. Controversy rages within the medical profession about the appropriate age for having a face-lift. The younger the skin and the more elasticity it has, the better and more long-lasting the results. For this reason, some surgeons are performing this operation on patients in their late thirties and early forties.

Other doctors feel it is wrong to encourage patients to have this type of elective surgery prematurely, and prefer to wait until people are in their late forties or their fifties and really have something to lift. Whether or when you should undergo a face-lift is a decision only you can make— but I hope you'll sift through the arguments on both sides and carefully weigh your own circumstances. There is no upper age limit, though—you can have a lift in your eighties as long as you are in good health.

Contrary to the "nip and tuck" mystique, a face-lift is *surgery* in the truest sense of the word, and a relatively long procedure at that. You'll need a complete physical examination before the operation can take place. As with any surgery, there are certain conditions that make you a high risk candidate. They include high blood pressure, heart disease, diabetes, kidney disease, and anemia.

Your surgeon must also know if you are taking any medication. Finally, be prepared to discuss your psychological reasons for wanting a face-lift. If you're looking for a cure-all or miracle, the truly ethical doctor will gently dissuade you from spending a large amount of money and time on what can only be a big letdown, and will recommend counseling instead of—or perhaps in addition to—surgery.

The operation takes upward of two hours, depending on exactly what procedures you are undergoing. As with blepharoplasty, a face-lift is usually done under local anesthetic and sedation. Both the operation and recovery period are quite painless.

The face-lift is one of the oldest forms of plastic surgery, although techniques have improved dramatically. The traditional lift involves stretching the skin of the face up and back from the jaw, toward the temples, and snipping off the excess. This can give a tight, masklike appearance to your face.

Many surgeons now prefer to use a procedure called SMAS-Platysma face-lift. In this operation, the underlying muscles and connective tissues are tightened and lifted along with the skin. The name comes from the two platysma muscles, which stretch from under the chin to the collarbone. The doctor shortens and repositions these and other muscles, then refits the skin snugly over them. If necessary, the doctor might also suction out underlying fatty deposits. This type of lift lasts longer and looks more natural than simply redraping the skin over the same old foundation.

The incisions are made under your chin, in front of and behind your ears, and along your hairline. Fortunately, it is not necessary to shave your head. After the operation, a dressing will be put on your face and left for a couple of days. You might experience a little tightness due to swelling, but you should not be in any real discomfort. Lie quietly for this immediate postoperative period.

After the bandages are off, it will take about another ten to fourteen days for the swelling and bruising to subside. The stitches will be removed during this time. In the month or so following your surgery, you should avoid strenuous exercise and sleep flat, without a pillow. As with all the procedures discussed so far, avoid the sun for at least three months.

Two weeks after your surgery, you should be ready to go out into the world with your new, youthful face. Only the fine scars in front of your ears will be visible, and only your hairdresser will know! But it's easy to camouflage these marks with makeup, or rearrange your hair over them until they fade.

THE PRICE OF YOUTH

Because most plastic surgery is elective and performed for cosmetic reasons, health-insurance plans rarely cover it. In some instances—such as when you need a blepharoplasty because drooping skin is obscuring your vision—you probably can get an insurance company to pay. There's a consolation prize: As long as a *doctor* performs the cosmetic procedure, the expense is tax deductible.

It may also surprise you to know that, according to statistics, about half of the cosmetic surgeries in recent years were performed on people with incomes of under $25,000 annually. Apparently, cost is not a deterrent to those whose minds are made up! In case you're wondering if you can afford cosmetic surgery, here is a tally of estimated fees:

Procedure	Price Range
Collagen Implants	$50–$200 per shot
Dermabrasion	$300–$2,500
Chemical Peel	$300–$2,500
Blepharoplasty	$600–$4,000
Face-lift	$2,000–$8,000

I know these prices are extremely wide-ranging, but that's because they vary so drastically from region to region, and from doctor to doctor. As in any profession, there are cut-rate operators: You can get a quickie, flat-rate face-lift, just as you can get a quickie, flat-rate divorce. But if someone makes a mistake on your face, you have no place to hide. This is one area where I urge you to shop around and get the best possible operation—even if it means paying more.

PART FIVE

THE MAKEOVERS

The women on the following pages are not professional models. They are from all walks of life and range in age from twenty-eight to seventy-two. Their only common traits are that they all have silver-gray hair and possess the kind of gusto for life that makes a woman sparkle with beauty at any age. I have included brief profiles about each because I'm sure you'll see yourself in at least one or two of them. There's no better inspiration!

The before-and-after photographs were taken in exactly the same location, with identical lighting, no more than two hours apart. I asked each woman to come with clean hair and face, and all were photographed *exactly* as they were when they walked through the door.

Then I called in our team of La Costa hair, skin, and makeup artists to teach each woman how she could look her very best. We wrought no miracles. We didn't play any tricks. No coloring or perming was done—although I did do some hair cutting. We ordered no plastic surgery and did not set out to change anyone's looks drastically.

So what did we do?

We simply used the resources available to everyone—hairstyling, cosmetics, wardrobe—to help each woman enhance and express her personal style.

In describing what we did to each, I won't go into a detailed, blow-by-blow account of every stroke of eye shadow or every flick of the tail comb. The techniques used have already been described in the preceding chapters. Instead, I'll tell you each model's specific problems and how I adapted my basic principles to make them work for her.

Some of the women shown have wrinkles; some have sun damage or display other signs of aging. We could have retouched these out of the photographs. But that would have given you false expectations of beauty techniques *and* of yourself. It would have left you frustrated when you couldn't achieve those unrealistically flawless looks. These are real women, with the same beauty problems and bonuses as you—and I think they look beautiful just the way they are.

They clearly thought so too. All of us at La Costa noticed that even those women who felt self-conscious when the photographer took the "before" shots, stood a little straighter, held their heads more proudly, and smiled more broadly for the "after" shots. There is an almost palpable air of self-confidence and pride about a woman who knows she looks her best.

PAT LIONEL

"How do you say, 'I'm a housewife,' and make it sound wonderful?" asks fifty-eight-year-old Pat. Well, now she can say she's a cover girl, too. Pat was such a natural in front of the camera that we asked her to let us use her makeover picture on the cover of the book.

Pat believes in staying busy, optimistic, and "happy under my own skin." Part of her means to that end includes a delight in gardening. "I like to bring into my home beautiful things I've grown," she says. "If I lived in a climate like California's instead of Nevada's, I'd probably try my hand at orchids or something exotic."

She has an abundance of patience when it comes to cooking and entertaining. "I love small parties, parties for a hundred people, all of it!" She counteracts the effects of her culinary skills with regular swimming (the stationary bike remains untouched—boring!) but still claims to have "the world's biggest appetite. The only *real* way to be thin is to zip up your mouth!"

Pat keeps an even temper and pleasant disposition by adhering to the philosophy "live and let live." "People don't always do things your way, even the ones who are close to you. One day I was explaining something to my five-year-old son, and said, 'I tried my best.' 'But Mommy, maybe *your* best wasn't the best thing!' he said. I'll always remember that."

But Pat's "best" when it comes to style suits her beautifully. "I don't do anything special about my looks. I've always worn a simple makeup style and have stayed a pastel person. Any color is fine as long as it's soft, although sometimes I'll try red without knowing why!

"My hair is a very unusual color—pale platinum. People are always asking me what coloring I use. I was fair as a child, but as I grew older, my hair turned light brown, and I streaked it, then went all blond. Finally, I noticed that my roots were a more interesting shade than the rest of my hair, so I let it all grow out. I'm so pleased! I don't have to do anything to it at all!"

PAT LIONEL

HAIR ANALYSIS
Texture: Medium-fine and wavy
Condition: Normal
Percentage of Silver: Seventy-five

FACE ANALYSIS
Skin Condition: Normal to dry
Wrinkles: Moderate around the eyes
Sun Damage: Patchy tan

COLOR PALETTE: Cool

BEAUTY BONUSES: Good skin, beautifully shaped mouth

AREA TO TROUBLESHOOT: Square, angular face

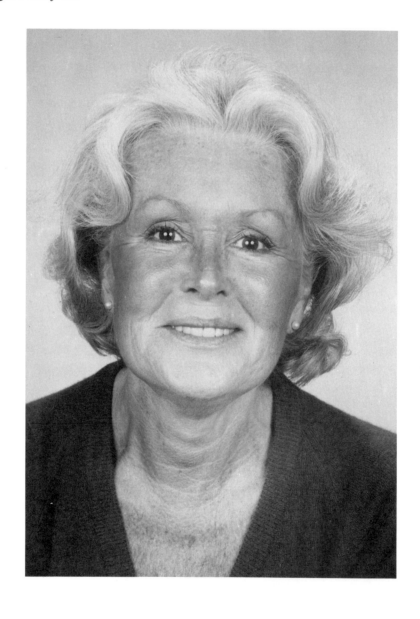

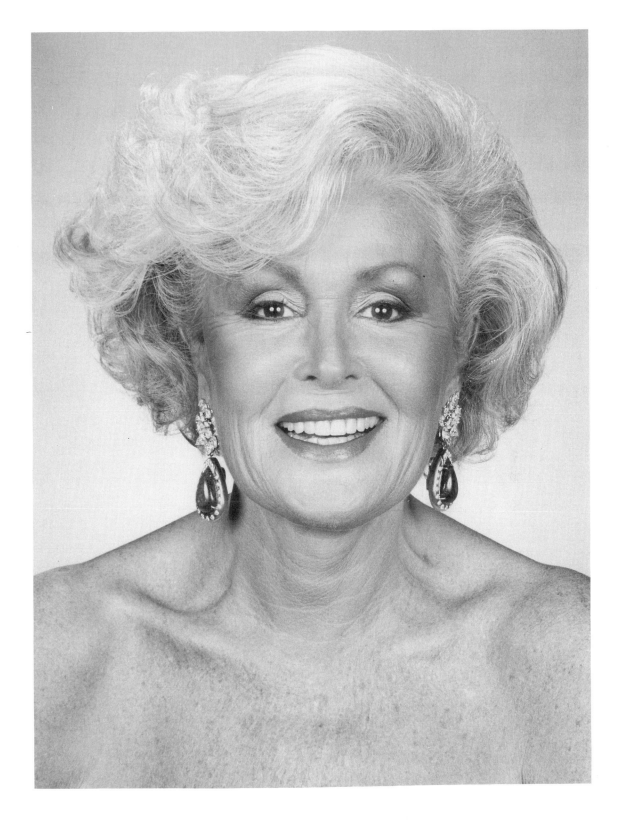

PAT LIONEL'S MAKEOVER

Pat's naturally fair hair has silvered sensationally. The transition from blond to silver has been a cinch. Her length and natural wave were just right. I simply gave her hair new direction and swept it to one side to soften the angular lines of her face. The flirty bangs are very feminine.

To get the shape, I set it in medium rollers in the direction of the movement. When it was dry, I had Pat bend forward while I brushed it out. Then she flipped her head back and it simply fell into place. A spritz of spray held it there.

We dotted light rose concealer on the bridge of Pat's nose and blended it to cover her patchy tan. Beige foundation and a dusting of translucent powder gave a matte, nighttime finish.

Because we were going for a glamorous, evening look, we got busy with the contour brush. We wielded a taupe powder on the widest part of her jaw to slim it down, and on the outer edge of her temples to mute the angularity of her face.

We created more defined cheekbones by using the same taupe contour powder under her cheekbones and up toward her temples. Her natural line got a swatch of *slightly* irridescent raspberry blush.

We filled out Pat's fine, light eyebrows with a taupe pencil, using feathery strokes. The start of sensational eyes—pearly, shell-pink highlighter. We used smoked navy shadow in the crease to contour, and swept it up and out a little. Charcoal liner and soft black mascara add drama.

Her cupid's bow was emphasized with a blue-red pencil and plum lipstick. A spot of gold blended on the center of her lower lip completes the look of nighttime dazzle.

Pat bares her beautiful shoulders in a strapless dress. The only accessories she needs are her own sumptuous earrings brought up from the vault (yes, they're real diamonds.) Pat is a picture of silver-gray glamour with a capital *G*.

LYNN KESSLER

Lynn, fifty-three, has led a life that sounds exciting to most of us. She was formerly a dancer, appearing in Las Vegas. She was also a "Copa Girl"—she danced at the fabulous Copacabana nightclub in New York City. It was at the Copa that she met her husband, who was managing another act that appeared there.

Now her husband operates a limousine business for the wealthy and glamorous, and Lynn is a real-estate agent whose turf is Beverly Hills. They retain an interest in show business, and, although they don't have much spare time because of the demands of work, they often go to the theater.

Lynn also likes to entertain at home. She feels that she has good relationships with people, because she tries to care for each person individually, and discover his or her special qualities.

But going out and entertaining are not priorities if it means sacrificing her own free time. "As I get older, I realize I want more time for myself," she says. She thinks her biggest problem is trying to do too much. "You've got to learn that each day can hold just so much—don't push too hard. When you try to take on too much, it only results in confusion, and nothing gets done. It's not that you have to slow down," she continues, "but you do have to achieve a balancing act."

For Lynn, that balancing act includes making sure she gets plenty of outdoor exercise. She considers walking to be an excellent means of keeping fit, and also likes cycling and playing tennis.

She occasionally considers covering her gray hair with color. "Sometimes it takes courage to keep it gray," she says. "But then the compliments come, and I decide to leave nature alone." Since her hair has turned gray, she avoids browns and favors more vibrant colors. She especially "adores black and white."

Lynn believes that "living, loving, and being at peace with yourself are what make life worthwhile. Life continues no matter how old you are."

LYNN KESSLER

HAIR ANALYSIS
Texture: Thick, wiry, curly
Condition: Normal, healthy
Percentage of Silver: One hundred at the sides, fifty on top, twenty-five at the back.

FACE ANALYSIS
Skin Condition: Normal
Wrinkles: Very few
Sun Damage: A couple of brown spots

COLOR PALETTE: Cool

BEAUTY BONUS: Enviably great skin

AREA TO TROUBLESHOOT: Narrow, heavy-lidded eyes, with almost no lashes.

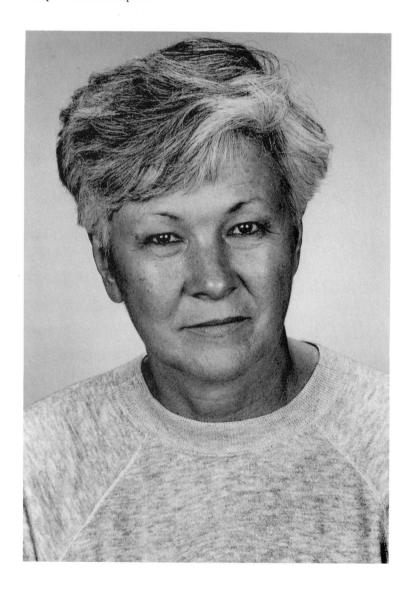

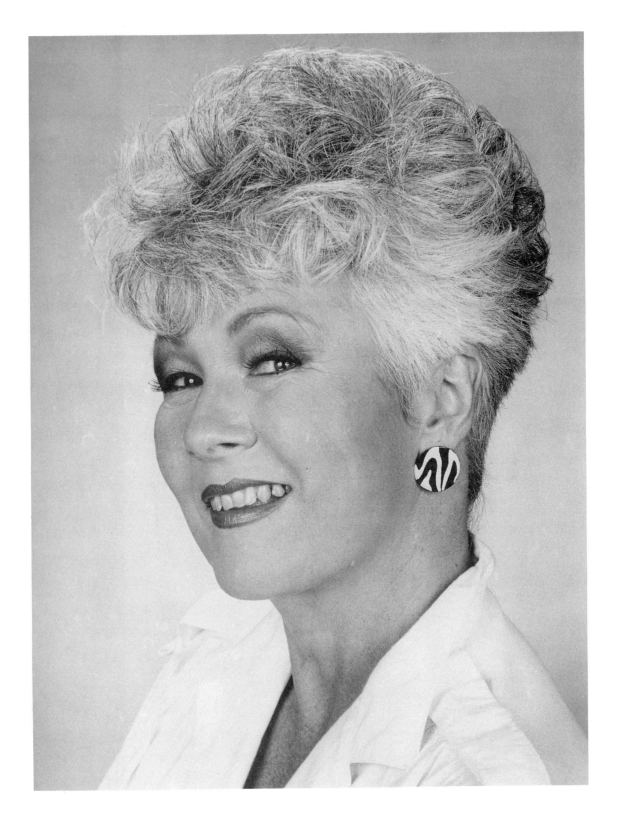

161

LYNN KESSLER'S MAKEOVER

Lynn's hair has gone silver in an extremely attractive way. I saw terrific possibilities in it, although she tends to wear it in an everyday, ho-hum style. It did not need reshaping, just a little trimming.

Mousse was spot-applied to the roots of her hair on the crown. I then "rough" blow-dried it and added some tousled curls on the crown with a curling iron. Strands were pulled down to draw attention to her eyes, and the back and sides were smoothed with a brush. It was all held in place with fast-drying sculpting spray. This style was much more spirited and energetic than Lynn's former style.

Lynn needed just a dab of bisque concealer on a couple of brown spots on her forehead and cheeks. After blending on a fair foundation, we fluffed on a translucent powder.

She has round, prominent cheeks, so we simply stroked a little heather blush on the "apple" of her cheeks.

Lynn's eyes presented a challenge. But we decided to celebrate rather than downplay what seem like beauty disadvantages. We created the illusion of an eyelid with a gunmetal-gray contour shadow in a distinct arc under her brow bone. A lighter-gray shadow was applied under the arc, and an oyster highlighter on the brown bone.

Lynn is a perfect candidate for false eyelashes. We used gray, natural-hair lashes applied in individual clumps to her upper lid. These, along with soft charcoal eye liner, opened her eyes right up.

Finally, we rectified her eyebrows, which had been overtweezed. In this instance, we drew in natural-looking brows with a brush and a taupe eyebrow powder. The end result was sparkly, seductive-looking eyes.

Lynn is lucky not to have wrinkles around her mouth. This allowed us the opportunity to line her lips just outside the natural line and give her rather thin mouth more fullness. Additionally, we shaped and defined her upper lip. We used a deep-rose-colored lipstick, because Lynn's teeth tended to have a yellowish tinge, and that would have been emphasized by bronze- or orange-tone lipstick.

Lynn's feeling about black and white is vindicated here. She displays a scene-stealing look in a simple white shirt and black-and-white earrings. The jewelry provides a bold point of focus without being overpowering.

SHANNON MADILL

At thirty-four, Shannon Madill is young to be sporting so much soft ash gray. But she absolutely loves her silver hair. "I'm uncomfortable with anything else," she says. "I've had to color it a couple of times for film parts when spraying it with color or wearing a wig didn't work, but then I couldn't wait to get it back to normal."

Shannon is literally a woman of action. As an actress who specializes in stunt work, she regularly falls off horses, gets into fights, and tumbles down stairs—it's enough to turn anyone gray! But the *tough* part of her work stems from the insecurity of show business.

"In this business, everything is a rollercoaster ride," says Shannon. "You need a strong sense of self, and the ability not to judge yourself or your success only by what is happening at the moment.

Energy may be her identifying mark, but she takes care not to burn herself out. "Sometimes, I become physically exhausted when I don't leave enough time for myself. I'm learning how to pull back and see life as a long-distance run, not a sprint," she says.

In between acting jobs, Shannon teaches aerobics classes and trains women with weights (for tone and definition, not bulk). She's even choreographed competition routines for women body builders. As you might imagine, Shannon is slim, fit, and well toned herself. She's a firm believer in using diet and exercise rather than cosmetic surgery to stay youthful.

To take a "break," Shannon goes horseback riding and bicycling in the mountains around Los Angeles. When she finally stops to rest, she likes to unwind with music: classical, jazz, blues.

Shannon also loves to go dancing with her stunt-man boyfriend. Then she likes to get all dressed up. "I work in a predominantly male field," she says. "You can't wear high heels if you're going to fall off a horse, so I really like to *dress* when I go out."

And that's when the compliments on her silver pour in. "People love my hair," she says. "With the right colors, it's very striking—I don't think it ages me at all. It's what you do with what you've got that makes the difference."

SHANNON MADILL

FACE ANALYSIS

Skin Condition: Normal, clear, with fine pores and good elasticity

Wrinkles: Some fine lines around her eyes

Sun Damage: Minimal, slightly uneven tan

HAIR ANALYSIS

Texture: Extremely fine, with some slight natural wave

Condition: Good, no perm or color

Percentage of Silver: Forty, with most lightness on top

COLOR PALETTE: True cool—no red or yellow highlights

BEAUTY BONUSES: Excellent skin, strong bone structure, beautifully shaped eyes and lips

AREAS TO TROUBLESHOOT: Undereye puffiness, a long face, and hard-to-style hair.

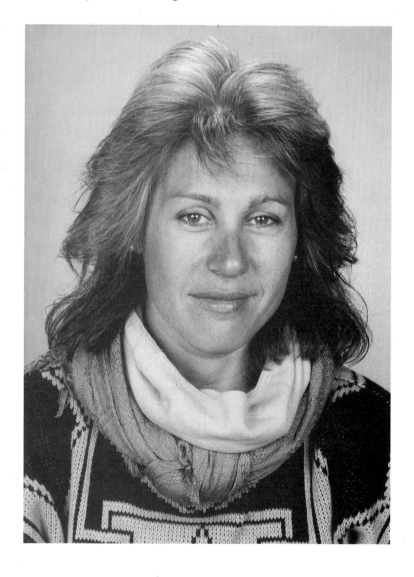

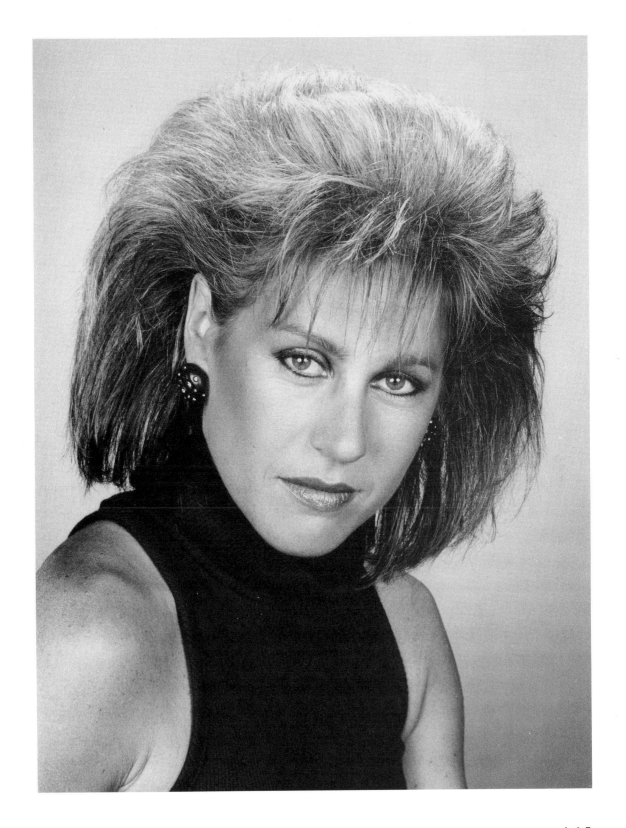

SHANNON MADILL'S MAKEOVER

Shannon's long hair was a little straggly, and the downward-flowing style did not flatter her face or make the most of her fine cheekbones. I blunt-cut it to shoulder level to create a thicker look.

After washing her hair, I applied a conditioner especially formulated for fine hair— a cream rinse would have made it limp and impossible to style.

I used styling gel rubbed into the roots with my fingertips to lift her hair away from her head and to add volume. I then styled it back off her face with a medium-size round brush and blow dryer on low heat. By taking her hair up and back, I counterbalanced Shannon's long face and revealed those stunning cheeks. Because her hair was so fine, I back-combed it slightly at the roots and held it in place with a mist of hair spray.

I pulled down some bangs which also helped reduce the length of her face and soften the look. I separated the strands into little wisps by using a blob of styling gel rubbed between my fingers. These wispy bangs can also camouflage horizontal lines on the forehead, although Shannon really didn't have many.

Shannon's beautiful face was a joy to work on. The first thing our La Costa makeup artists did was clean up her eyebrows by tweezing stragglers from the bridge of her nose.

Next we applied light rose-beige concealer in the crease *under* the puffiness beneath her eyes. We also used concealer on the lines from nose to mouth and to bring her suntanned nose into line with the rest of her face. It was all carefully blended with a damp sponge.

We used rose-beige foundation and set it with a dusting of translucent powder.

We defined her cheekbones with a soft cocoa contour powder applied under the bone and a lick of pink blush on the bone. They were blended together by buffing with a wide, fluffy brush.

Her nose needed slimming down, so we used the same cocoa contour powder on the sides of her nose.

Because I was aiming for a glamorous look, we gave Shannon's almond-shaped eyes our nighttime makeup: misty-pink highlighter over her entire lid, eggplant contour above the crease, clear blue accent with color concentrated in the outer corners, smudged charcoal liner rimming both upper and lower lids, soft black mascara. We filled in her brows with a gray pencil and brushed them into place.

Her lips are perfectly shaped, so we followed the natural line and colored with a lustrous true-pink lipstick. Just a spot of gold blended on her lower lip gave a pouty effect.

Only someone as fit as Shannon can carry off a dress with scooped-out shoulders the way she can. But thanks to her well-toned muscles (not a trace of upper-arm flab!) it looks sensational. The high collar defines her good jawline; heavy ceramic earrings complete the outfit for a look that's bold . . . *sexy*. Shannon went from tomboy to glamour girl in less than an hour!

CAREY SIMON

Carey's silver hair has always made her feel special. "It's been salt-and-pepper since I was about sixteen," says Carey, now thirty-six.

She finds that being prematurely gray encourages her to avoid drab colors and take special pains to have a good, stylish haircut—very important for her busy life-style. Carey is typical of many women her age—she opted for establishing her career before becoming a mother in her mid-thirties. She was the editor of a magazine that is placed in hotel rooms for guests, but left her job to work freelance when she had a child, who is now two years old.

"I'm a fabulous mother," she says. "I waited a long time to have my daughter. I was truly prepared to give of myself. I feel no conflict between motherhood and my career. I'm comfortable with the way things are."

Freelance work poses a unique problem for Carey. "When you work full time, you're forced to schedule things carefully. But when you're on your own, you think there's all the time in the world. Not true!" When she does have a little time, she spends it reading or doing essential shopping.

She finds that she is not really motivated to find time for a formal exercise program. She occasionally does the Jane Fonda Workout, which she has on video tape, but only when she's in the mood.

For fun, Carey likes to go out for a casual dinner. She and her husband enjoy trying new restaurants. They also entertain friends at home, and her husband shares the cooking. Once a year, they throw a big chili party with a guest list of over a hundred people. Carey's basic philosophy? "Stop and look around you," she advises. "Appreciate life as it happens."

CAREY SIMON

HAIR ANALYSIS
Texture: Thick, straight, and slightly wiry
Condition: Excellent
Percentage of Silver: Fifty, evenly sprinkled throughout her hair

FACE ANALYSIS
Skin Condition: Slightly oily, but fine-textured
Wrinkles: Some around the eyes; few early signs of aging
Sun Damage: Minimal; scattered freckles

COLOR PALETTE: Warm, but with yellow rather than red tones predominating

BEAUTY BONUS: Glossy, healthy hair

AREAS TO TROUBLESHOOT: Sallow skin, dark undereye circles

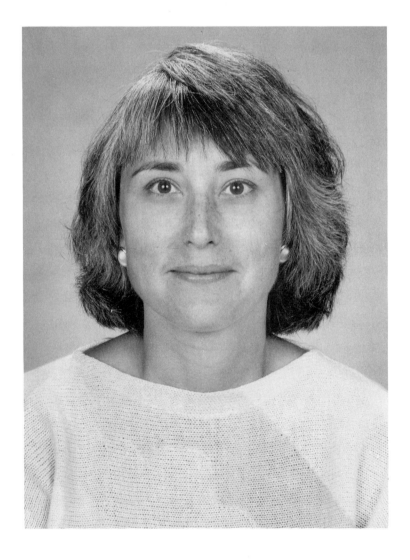

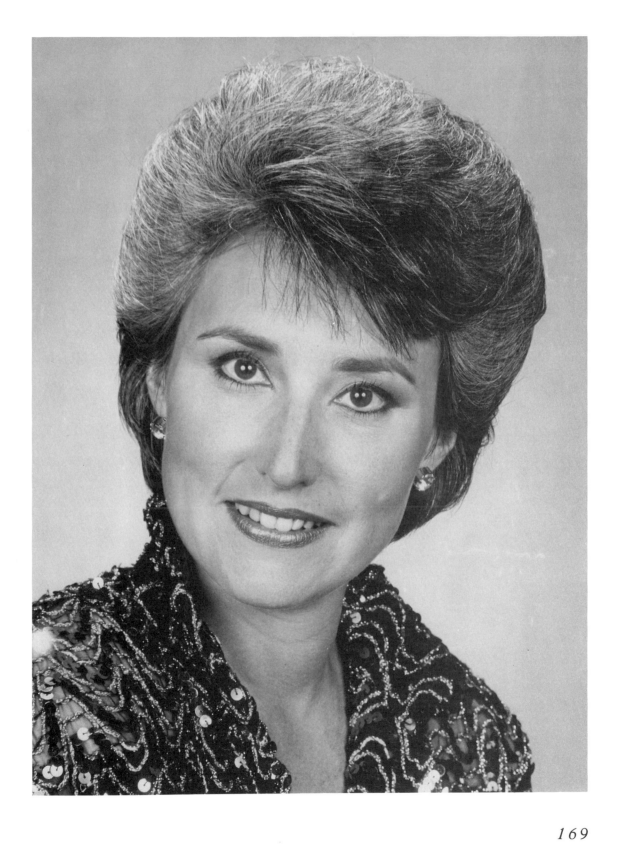

CAREY SIMON'S MAKEOVER

Although Carey's hair was well cut in a contemporary bob, the style really was not flattering to her. She has an extremely square face, and wearing her hair cropped at chin level only accentuated that. I scissored her hair into a shorter, layered style, with a little hair showing just below her ears to soften her jawline.

Her hair needed little conditioning. I combed a handful of mousse through it to achieve fullness before blow drying it, and then swept it back smoothly to enhance the attractive growth pattern of her silver.The sideswept bangs are soft and feminine, and dramatically play up her eyes.

Carey's eyebrows were straight and heavy, and needed tweezing from the undersides to form a gentle arch.

We took care of her freckles and undereye darkness with ivory concealer.

To counteract her sallowness, we used sand foundation, which added the red tones she was lacking. Loose powder fluffed on and dusted off helped avoid shine from her oily skin. Coral powder blush on her cheekbones further warmed her cheeks.

Carey has extremely pretty, widely spaced brown eyes. Because her eyes are so far apart, the bridge of her nose looks broad. Above the creases of her lids, *contour* eyeshadow brought well into the inner corners has a slenderizing effect. We emphasized her upward-slanting eyes by sweeping sable eye liner up and out just a little.

In keeping with her coloring, Carey has brown-toned lips. We brightened them with a clear coral lipstick. You'll notice that her lips tend to curve down; we lined her upper lip just short of the corner of her mouth, and extended the lower line a little for counterbalance.

I wanted to keep Carey's bright, sparkling beauty at all costs. Even though I had her made up for nighttime, we wielded the cosmetics *subtly* for a "clean" look, not a heavy, overly sophisticated one.

Her glittery black-and-silver top and diamond earrings perfectly complement her black-and-silver hair! The upturned collar and deep V neckline further slim down her square face.

Carey went from girlish to womanly without losing any of her innate, fresh charm.

PAT McCORMICK

Pat McCormick has done something no one else has ever done. At consecutive Olympic games—in Helsinki in 1952 and Melbourne in 1956—she won gold medals in both platform and springboard diving events. This back-to-back, double-double achievement earned her a place in the Olympic Hall of Fame in 1986 and an accolade from the United States Olympic Committee as "the finest women's diver in the history of the games."

As if that weren't enough, Pat went ahead and raised a daughter, Kelly, who took the silver medal for diving in the 1984 Olympics in Los Angeles. During those games, Pat was an official spokesperson assigned to protocol.

This remarkable woman is now a motivational speaker. She obtained a degree in business, and travels around the country addressing both schoolchildren and business people on the subject of success—achieving it and maintaining it. Her philosophy is, "Set a goal. When you reach it, replace it. But you must nurture yourself also—maintain a balance. What good is it if you reach your goals by slighting yourself?" She has a series of audio tapes on the subject, and is currently writing a book.

At the age of fifty-five, Pat has long since given up competing in diving contests, but she still finds time for plenty of physical activity. She maintains her level of fitness and her trim figure with half an hour of swimming and an hour of aerobics every morning. "This is serious work, and I don't consider it fun!" she says. For fun, she rides horseback, plays golf, and skis, depending on the season. She also pilots a small plane.

Pat's leisure time is mostly spent outdoors, but she also thinks "dressing up is terrific," and loves to go out dancing or to the movies.

Her years in the outdoors have taken their toll on Pat's hair and skin. But her bubbly personality, infectious smile, and sparkling eyes give her a youthful beauty that no amount of sun damage can obscure. "Silver hair is not a symbol of old age," she says. "Age is a state of mind. I love where I am right now, and I'm looking forward to the next forty years."

PAT McCORMICK

HAIR ANALYSIS
Texture: Very thin and fine, with a little natural wave
Condition: Extremely dry and damaged from sun and chlorine
Percentage of Silver: One hundred, but "tinted" slightly yellow by the sun and pool water

FACE ANALYSIS
Skin Condition: Very dry
Wrinkles: Many around the eyes
Sun Damage: Extreme

COLOR PALETTE: Warm

BEAUTY BONUSES: Well-shaped mouth and excellent, white teeth

AREAS TO TROUBLESHOOT: Hair and skin "fried" by the elements

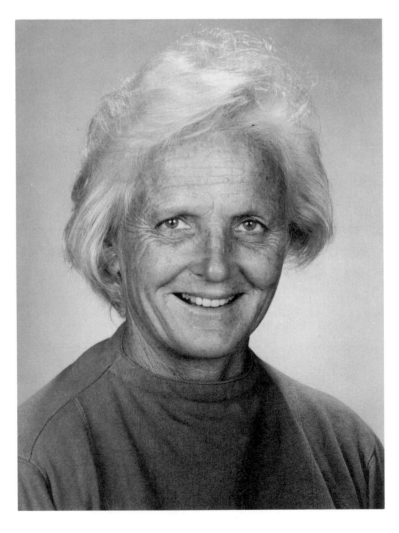

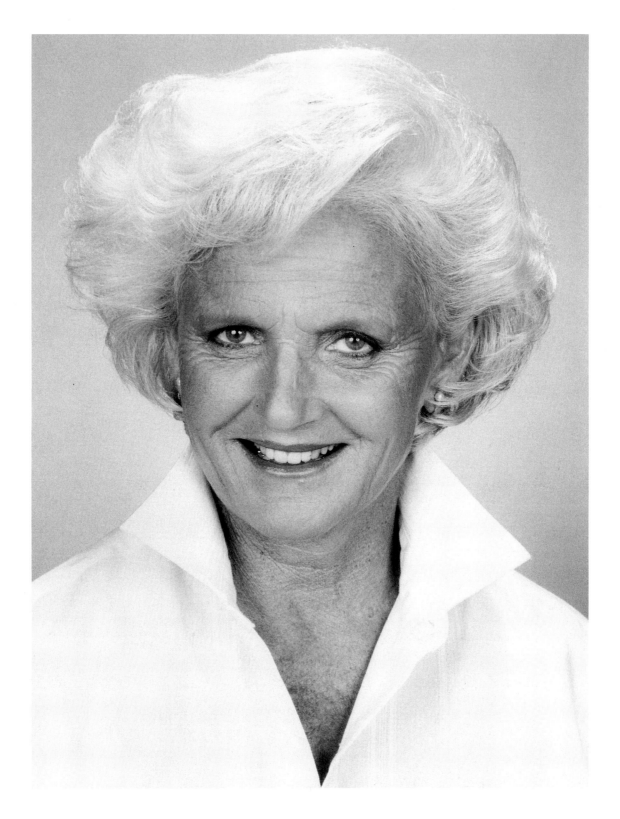

PAT McCORMICK'S MAKEOVER

I gave Pat's hair a chemical rinse to remove traces of chlorine and recommended that she occasionally use a shampoo such as UltraSwim.

Pat's basic haircut is fine, but she tends to wear it in a neglected "nondo." I showed her that it only took ten minutes to dress it in an equally unstudied but more youthful style. I used an alcohol-free styling gel and a blow dryer on the low setting to style it. The upswept sides detract from the lines around her eyes, and the deep, soft waves reflect the light, making her hair look shiny and healthy.

Pat is a prime example of someone whose life story is etched on her face. She has many lines around her eyes from squinting into the sun, and has uneven pigmentation—also from the sun—and parched skin from years of being outdoors and in chlorinated pools. Her skin needs moisturizing and more moisturizing. We recommended a collagen-enriched cream that will help temporarily plump up lines.

Beige-tan concealer was blended under her eyes, on the bridge of her nose, and on brown spots.

We chose to go with a foundation that was a shade lighter than her skin tone: Her deep tan tends to draw attention to her lines. In this case—although it is not usually recommended—we took the foundation down her neck a little way and faded it into her natural skin tone. Why? Because we had slightly altered the color of her face and didn't want to leave a line around her jaw.

Pat should forgo loose powder, as it can settle in creases and create a caked look. We just gave her some cheek color, with a deep apricot blush brushed on the cheekbones that was perfect on her tanned complexion. A slight dusting of tan contour powder on her temples and under her jawline gave her round face more definition.

Notice that Pat has almost no eyebrows. After talking it over with our whole team, I decided to leave them that way, because it looks natural on her and because we thought that to draw some in would call attention to the lines around her eyes.

By making her eyes up in earthy tones, as for hooded eyes, the deep-olive contour eye shadow had the effect of opening them up.

Pat has a well-shaped mouth and excellent white teeth, made all the better with coral lip color.

Although Pat is now a businesswoman, her overall look is still sporty. She is stylish and snappy in this man's cotton shirt with the collar flipped up. The neat, pearl-stud earrings give her outfit the finishing touch. In turn, we gave this "golden girl" just a finishing touch of sophistication.

KATHERYN FRANKEL

A few years ago, Katheryn Frankel was taken by a friend for a ride in a hot-air balloon. She fell in love with the experience and promptly signed up for lessons. After getting her pilot's license, this self-proclaimed "self-starter" began her own ballooning business, taking other adventurers up into the wild blue yonder. But what had been a wonderful pastime lost some of its sparkle when her life became clogged up with business minutiae, so Katheryn returned to the status of amateur ballooner.

Now she works as Director of Guest Services at La Costa, mixing and mingling with the spa's visitors. She gets plenty of compliments from them on her stunning gray hair. "People ask me how I get it this color," she says. "And I tell them, genes. It started to turn white when I was sixteen, and I've never felt any need at all to change the color."

Katheryn likes clothes, since her job keeps her in the public eye at this glamorous resort, she always puts her outfits together carefully. Because of her hair color she tends to stick to bright shades, and she finds it best to avoid yellow and gray. She loves classical music, and her idea of a terrific night out is to dress up and go to a concert.

It's important to Katheryn to fit these special times into her life. "I'm a compulsive person; I have trouble relaxing," she says. "I enjoy being alive. I enjoy the things I do. But I need time to myself, and feel cheated if I don't get it."

One of the things she does for herself is maintain a regular exercise program. She has worked out a personal routine that includes light weights for muscle definition, and aerobics on a rebounder for cardiovascular conditioning and weight control.

KATHERYN FRANKEL

HAIR ANALYSIS
Texture: Thick, strong, with some natural wave
Condition: Healthy
Percentage of Silver: One hundred on top, seventy-five on the sides

FACE ANALYSIS
Skin Condition: Very dry, but blemish-free
Wrinkles: Fine network around the eyes
Sun Damage: Minimal

COLOR PALETTE: Cool

BEAUTY BONUS: Classic oval face

AREAS TO TROUBLESHOOT: Wide nose, unflattering hairstyle

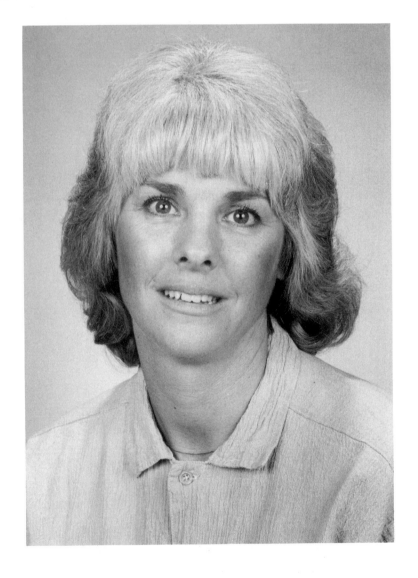

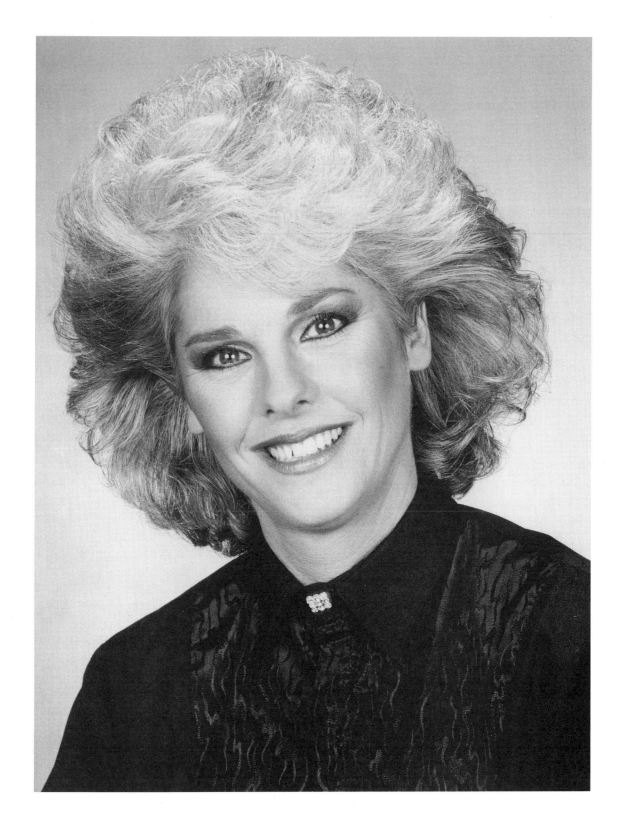

KATHERYN FRANKEL'S MAKEOVER

Because of her busy schedule, Katheryn wanted to keep her medium-length hair in a simple cut. I thought the style was a little dowdy, and that her straight, heavy bangs were too childish for a sophisticated woman. Without cutting it, I set her hair loose and dressed it in a much more grown-up look, using styling mousse and medium-size hot rollers. The sideswept bangs show off the beautiful color to better advantage, and the fullness at the sides accentuates her face, making it seem more delicate.

Her eyebrows needed work. Not only were they too close to her eyes; they were also dark and heavy and contrasted sharply with the very light hair framing her brow. We tweezed them into a finer arch and lightened them one shade with eyebrow bleach to bring her hair and face into better harmony. (Katheryn should have her brows professionally bleached about every six weeks. It's a tricky procedure that's best not tried at home.)

We recommended that Katheryn drink several glasses of water a day to see a rapid improvement in her dry skin. In the meantime, we applied moisturizer before we made her up.

Her cheeks were slightly ruddy, but were evened out with two different foundation colors—porcelain on the ruddy areas and medium beige on the rest—blended directly on her skin with a damp sea sponge. We did not use powder, as her skin was so dry.

We sculpted cheekbones by brushing taupe contour shadow directly under the bone and up to her temples. Then we emphasized the shape of Katheryn's face by shading just under her chin with the same contour powder.

To give the illusion of making her wide nose look narrow, we wielded the contour brush on the sides of her nose from the bridge to the tip. The shading needed careful blending with a clean brush.

We continued the illusion by bringing the smoked navy eye shadow we used above the crease of her lid well into the inner corners of her eyelids.

Katheryn has pale lips, which almost fade away to nothing. Furthermore, the shape of her upper lip lacks definition. We blended a little concealer around her mouth to blur the natural line before drawing in a more shapely cupid's bow with a well-sharpened blue-red pencil and fuschia lipstick.

The black blouse Katheryn is wearing is actually a man's dress shirt—borrowing from the boys is a clever fashion trick. The only jewelry she needs is a simple rhinestone pin at the throat. It provides the edge that's needed to spark her appearance, but without fussiness. The style she projects is an extremely cosmopolitan evening look that can take her to the symphony or a disco.

BEVERLY DINI

In common with many of her peers, at the age of fifty, Beverly has recently become a single woman again. "I suppose I feel a little vulnerable now that I'm on my own," she says, "but I think women are better able to handle these things today. We seem somehow larger and stronger."

She may be single, but she's not alone. Much of Beverly's time is absorbed in her two daughters and her son. Also, she enjoys company immensely, and loves to put on a special outfit and go out. She steers clear of the singles-bar scene, and prefers private clubs or sports-related events.

Her job of seven years also offers her plenty of opportunity to meet people. Beverly is the buyer for and manager of a gift shop. "I love my work, and have become completely involved in it," she says. "I wouldn't leave my job now even if I didn't have to work."

In her quiet times Beverly is a big reader. "I'm in a transitional phase, and find psychology books particularly interesting. I always seem to be learning something about myself," she says.

Right now, Beverly walks for exercise. But in keeping with her philosophy that it is important to branch out and try new activities, she is planning to learn to sail. She also admits to being a procrastinator, however, so who knows if she has started yet!

Beverly's hair, which is about 50 percent gray, only started to lighten about ten years ago. "If it had turned gray when I was thirty, I might have colored it," she admits. As it happens, she was thinking about having her hair frosted, when "nature did it for me." She is now perfectly content with her hair color, and even thinks "gray is so interesting; I get a lot of admiration."

BEVERLY DINI

HAIR ANALYSIS
Texture: Coarse and straight
Condition: Good
Percentage of Silver: Fifty—salt and pepper

FACE ANALYSIS
Skin Condition: Oily
Wrinkles: A few around the lips, but skin has retained a remarkably youthful texture
Sun Damage: Minimal

COLOR PALETTE: Warm

BEAUTY BONUSES: Excellent, healthy hair and skin

AREAS TO TROUBLESHOOT: Badly shaped eyebrows, slight overbite.

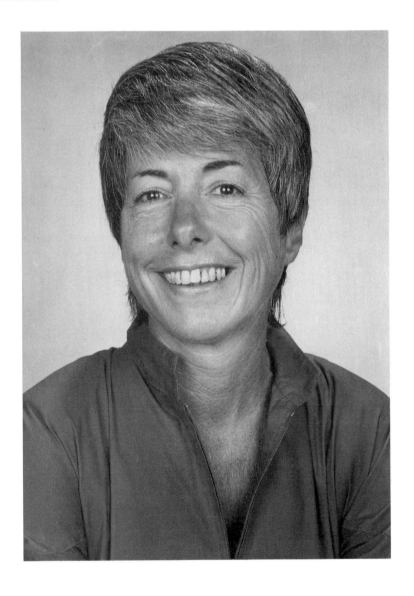

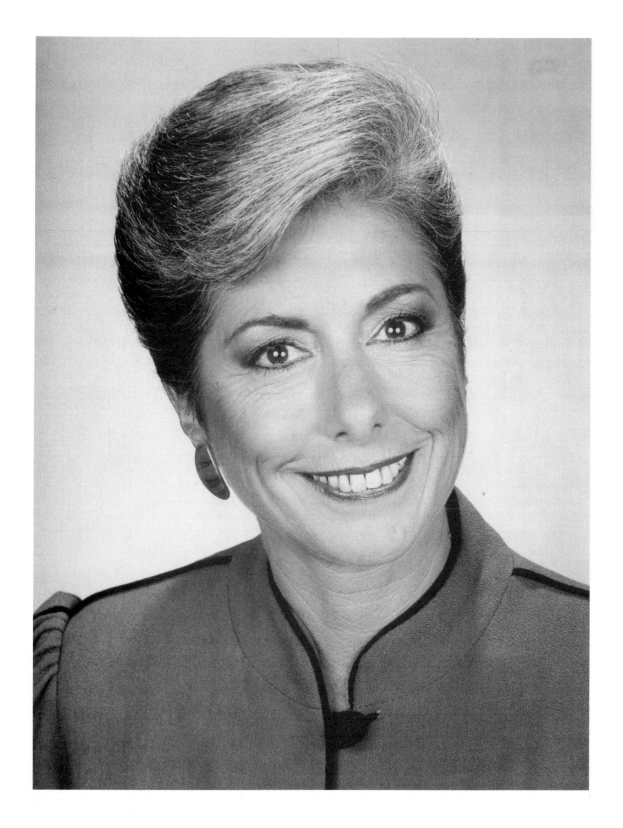

BEVERLY DINI'S MAKEOVER

Beverly loves her wash-and-go style. She has the type of hair that can be terrific in a simple cut. I simply trimmed it at the nape of her neck, as it was a little ragged and did not work with the high collars she likes to wear. Losing that back hair also gave her neck a more slender appearance.

When I experimented with combing her hair in different directions, I found that Beverly was not making the most of the growth pattern of her gray. Brushed over to her left, as she usually wore it, her hair had a salt-and-pepper look. But when I swept it over to the right, a deep wave of color was revealed that was much more distinct. Also, when I took the sides back instead of forward, her original, dark hair became apparent, and contrasted dramatically with the gray. This sleek, modern coif is the perfect complement for her hair.

Beverly's hair has a good deal of gold pigmentation, and her silver can take on a yellowish cast. I recommended that she use a semipermanent silver rinse to counteract it. In the meantime, I set her hair with Fancifull's White Minx Color Styling Mousse as a temporary solution.

Beverly has the type of oily skin that ages well. It needed only a dab of moisture lotion smoothed around her eyes and lips.

We used two different shades of water-based foundation: a lighter color, cream, in the center of her face, blended into a darker color, tan. This was to give an illusion of length to her rather round face.

We shaded under her cheekbones and from ear to ear under her chin with sepia contour powder to give the shape of her face extra definition.

We had words with Beverly over what she had done to her eyebrows: tweezed them into foreshortened horizontal commas. We showed her how to use a well-sharpened sable pencil to correct the problem. We feathered in a line along her brow bone and ended the "new" brow a quarter of an inch beyond the outer corner of her eyes. The arch looked more elegant.

Beverly had a wide space between her eyebrows and her lash line. After applying ivory highlighter as a base, we blended an olive eye shadow over her entire lid and took it up to the brow at the outer corners. This also makes her eyes look more open.

A fixative cream was used as a base on Beverly's lips, because she had some vertical lines around her mouth into which lip color can bleed.

To help counteract her slight overbite, we drew a line just outside her natural one to make her lower lips more full, and finished the makeup with a bronze lipstick.

Crisp and nonthreateningly businesslike is Beverly's style. The simply detailed suit she is wearing in the "after" picture has the same fit and familiarity as her outfit in the "before" picture, but with something added. The pleated sleeves give her shoulders a more confident set, and the buttoned-up neck covers her freckled chest. Contemporary earrings provide the finishing touch.

JANET NEWMAN

Janet, fifty-nine, is originally from the Midwest. She traveled to Los Angeles on her own in the forties, "when that wasn't such a common thing for a young woman to do."

She became a surgical nurse, a profession from which she retired three years ago. But retirement hasn't meant that she has become inactive—she now works as a buyer alongside her husband in the family-owned shoe and handbag business. "I think when a woman works, it is an incentive to look good. Keep your mind active; move your body," says Janet. "I feel like I'm twenty-five because I'm busy."

"Busy" seems an understatement. Janet and her husband are avid theatergoers, and also subscribe to the Los Angeles Philharmonic. They regularly entertain at home—either at barbecues or at sit-down dinners for eight. Furthermore, they occasionally take courses in current events at the local community college. "It's important to stimulate your mind," Janet says. She also plays the piano and loves art-gallery hopping.

On the physical side, Janet's chief form of exercise is walking, and she spends hours working in her garden. She also enjoys swimming, but does not actively pursue it.

Janet is justifiably proud of having lost fifty pounds and keeping it off. Her favorite foods are fresh fruits and vegetables—"I could live on salads," she says—and she avoids red meat.

During her career as a nurse, Janet assisted in cosmetic surgeries. She offers this advice: "If you decide on surgery, choose a board-certified plastic surgeon." She sees nothing wrong with seeking professional help to improve your appearance if you think you need it.

Personally, she favors "a program of preventive care—the sun can be devastating, so I always use a sunscreen and wear a hat for gardening—proper diet, exercise, and attitude. Attitude is all-important.

"I always try to look my best," she continues. "It gives me a lift. When you know you look good, you feel great! But it isn't practical to spend forty-five minutes on your hair and makeup in the morning. Ten minutes should be enough for every day." Janet admits to learning something from our makeover. She has vowed to start wearing blusher.

Janet used to frost her hair, but thinks it is prettier now that she has let it remain at its natural 80 percent silver. "I'm quite comfortable with it," she says. "Besides, some women spend hundreds of dollars to get this look!"

JANET NEWMAN

HAIR ANALYSIS
Texture: Coarse, wiry, naturally curly
Condition: Normal
Percentage of Silver: Eighty

FACE ANALYSIS
Skin Condition: Good, slightly coarse texture
Wrinkles: Some around the eyes
Sun Damage: Very little

COLOR PALETTE: Warm, but very muted

BEAUTY BONUSES: Chiseled cheekbones, dramatic eyes

AREA TO TROUBLESHOOT: Thin, shapeless lips

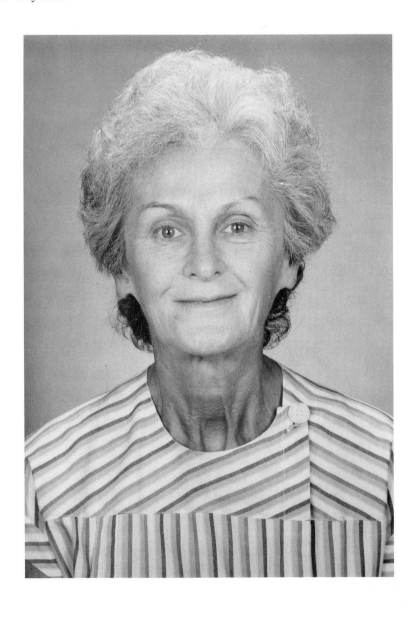

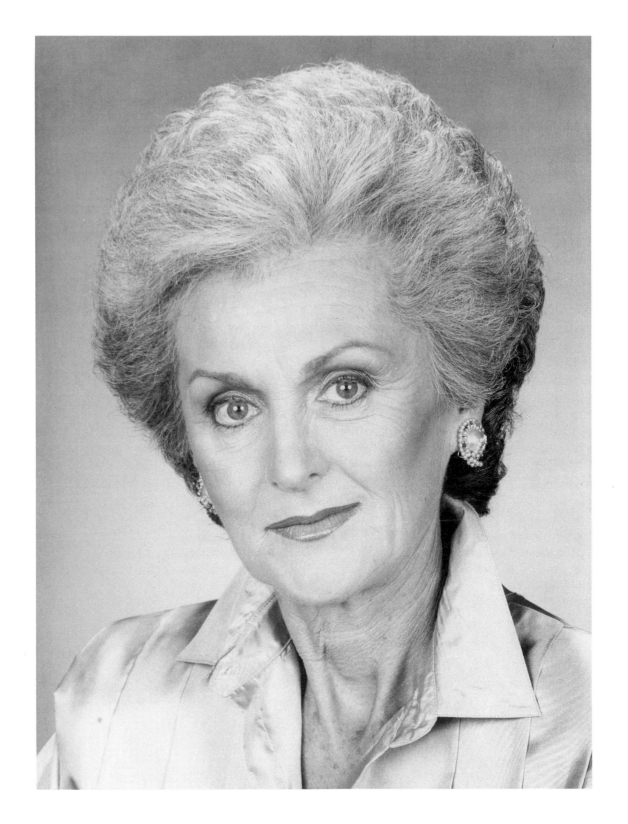

JANET NEWMAN'S MAKEOVER

There was nothing drastic I needed to do to Janet's hair. It is slightly uncontrollable, as her natural curl has relaxed a little with time. I recommended that she use a good cream rinse to tame it and make it manageable.

Her cut was flattering, the back-swept top accented her fine eyes and high forehead. I simply energized her look by dressing her hair into a fuller, more polished version of her basic style. I set it in big, loose pincurls while we worked on her face. This truly was a case of doing minimal enhancing.

All that sunblock and hat-wearing has paid off for Janet; her skin is excellent. We used a small amount of concealer on isolated brown spots; a soft peach foundation did the job of evening out the color and refining the texture.

Janet has the chiseled cheekbones that are the envy of everyone. She needed no contouring; we simply warmed her cheeks with salmon blusher stroked over the bone.

Janet's eyes are her most dramatic feature. They are large, with deep sockets. We used a rich brandy in the crease from the bridge of her nose to the outer corner of the eyes. The thick but not-too-dark brown liner on her upper and lower lids made her eyes look rounder.

We penciled in less-ragged eyebrows, taking care to not make them too thick or heavy, as her face is delicate. To get the effect we wanted, we used two colors of pencil: light brown and blond.

Her lips were extremely thin and shapeless. We drew a distinct line outside her natural line on both the top and bottom lips. Then we filled them in with a rich coral lipstick. You can see that this technique can look very natural if skillfully applied.

Janet is typical of those women whose skin and hair have lightened in harmony, giving her an almost ethereal look. She is at her best when she sticks to soft colors and textures. Her silky, petal-soft shirt and pearl earrings are just right.

Janet has a somewhat sinewy throat area. The high, round neckline in her "before" picture draws immediate attention to it. On the other hand, the shirt neckline with upturned collar in the second photograph is far more flattering. The large clip-on earrings help camouflage her large earlobes. The overall effect is one of understated elegance.

JUNE CAIN-MILLER

Readers in southern California will undoubtedly recognize June as the hostess of a television talk show broadcast daily on a local station. June, aged fifty-four, is convinced that her career and life turned around after her hair went gray. "I'm noticed more, and I feel unique," she says. "People refer to me as the woman with gray hair. Before it was 'the brunette,' but half the women in the room were 'the brunette"!

June grew up in Pennsylvania, in a family of twelve children. "I was lucky to grow up in such a large family," she says. "I believe my personality was greatly influenced by it. It taught me to be direct, to go one on one." Perhaps it is this trait that makes her such a good talk-show hostess.

Although June is widowed now, she has three children and a granddaughter, all of whom live with her. She loves having her family around her. "You can afford to be yourself because you are assured of unconditional love. Everything and everyone else is gravy. I suppose my biggest problem is not being able to let go," she says.

Between her friends and her church, she has a full social life, but she is not interested in dating right now. She is sure that will come later, when she has achieved her personal goals.

June has been a sports fan all her life, both as a participator and a spectator. At school she played hockey and basketball, although she is only five-feet two. And she was a cheerleader "way back when." She follows football passionately—her favorite team is still the Philadelphia Eagles, although she admits to a growing affection for the Los Angeles Raiders.

When it comes to beauty, June believes that "skin is your greatest asset. It tells all, and you should give it more care than any other aspect of your beauty routine. Cleansing is all-important; I couldn't sleep if I hadn't removed my makeup." She thinks that diet, exercise, and rest are every bit as vital as cleansing and moisturizing. As for cosmetic surgery, "I love the idea. I'm going to have it myself someday."

Because her job puts her in the public eye, June dresses up most of the time. She finds her gray hair a bonus in this respect, as "I can wear any color with it; everything looks good."

JUNE CAIN-MILLER

HAIR ANALYSIS
Texture: Thick and wiry
Condition: Extremely dry
Percentage of Silver: Seventy-five

FACE ANALYSIS
Skin Condition: Dry
Wrinkles: Deeply etched laugh lines around the eyes
Sun Damage: Moderate

COLOR PALETTE: Cool

BEAUTY BONUS: Well-shaped lips

AREAS TO TROUBLESHOOT: Asymmetrical nose

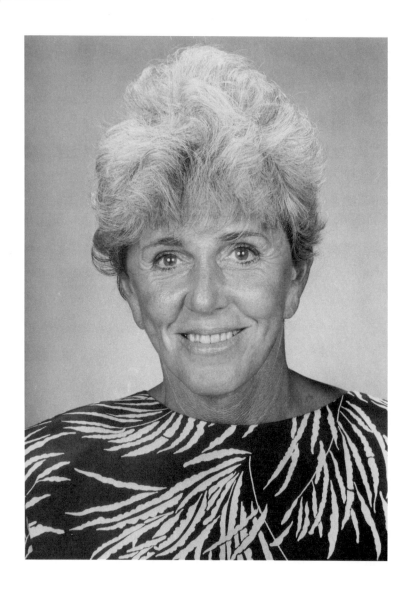

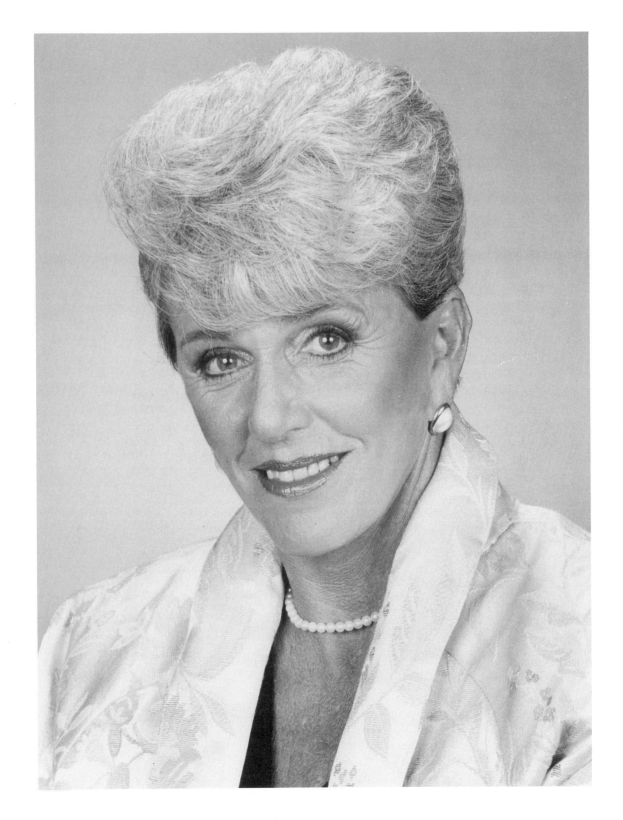

JUNE CAIN-MILLER'S MAKEOVER

I treated June's hair with an oil-based deep conditioner formulated for dry hair, and recommended she do the same on a monthly basis. This will give it shine and manageability.

Her short cut needed only to be trimmed at the sides and back. A dab of styling lotion kept her hair smoothly in place. I left the length and fullness on top, but tamed her unruly curls into a more sleek, sophisticated style by blow drying them.

All that attention to her skin has really been worthwhile for June; the texture of her skin is good. It looked fine with a sheer layer of foundation (no powder; it would settle in the lines around her eyes), and with pink blush on her cheekbones.

So as not to draw attention to her laugh lines, we kept June's eye makeup to subtle smoke contour and lilac highlighter. We used wine eye liner, gently smudged.

June's biggest beauty challenge is that her nose is asymmetrical. There is nothing wrong with having a quirky feature like this; it adds individuality to a face. But for occasions when she wants to create a balanced look, we showed her how to use a little makeup magic. To even it out, we used a darker foundation on the right side of her nose and a lighter color on the left, applied with swabs. All was carefully blended with a damp sea sponge, so as not to leave any noticeable lines.

June has a well-shaped mouth, but we made her top lip slightly fuller with raspberry lip liner and lipstick.

On camera, June has an image to project. She appears cool, confident, and in charge. We show off her softer side with a pretty print brocade jacket in pastel pinks and mauves. Pearls complete the picture.

MARTHA GRESHAM

This woman is a dynamo! Martha has been in business as an interior designer for thirty years. She started out in the Palm Desert area of California designing condos. Now she works mainly on the California "Riviera," covering the exclusive communities of Newport Beach, San Clemente, and Laguna. As the head of a company of nine people, Martha designs large office buildings and entire commercial units. "I love what I do, and that keeps me young," she says.

One of Martha's most exciting projects was saving a San Juan Capistrano landmark called the Forster Mansion. "I sold my home to finance this project," she says. "It took about six months, and I lived that restoration! I was completely involved in every aspect. It was worth it. Another year and it would have been gone, but now it is beautiful." Martha not only had the satisfaction of saving this fine old building; she also works out of it.

She is now pursuing another dream. Martha would like to design a health spa. "I love the idea of a spa," she says. "It is not just terrific physically, it also helps you mentally and spiritually." She already has the perfect site picked out—by the ocean in San Clemente. She would like to run the spa once it is completed.

Martha is deeply involved in charity work. She supports the arts in particular—she thinks they are in need because of government cutbacks—and she is on the board of directors of the local Master Chorale. She thinks her energy and love of people are her best attributes. "As you get older, you either gear up or slide downhill," she says.

At fifty-eight, Martha's hair is pure silver. "I remember my grandmother's having hair like this, and I love it," she says. She has never thought of coloring it. In fact, she is quite proud of "what I've done with what I have."

MARTHA GRESHAM

HAIR ANALYSIS
Texture: Exceptionally thin and fine
Condition: Normal
Percentage of Silver: One hundred

FACE ANALYSIS
Skin Condition: Fine-pored, with good texture
Wrinkles: Some loss of elasticity
Sun Damage: Some brown spots

COLOR PALETTE: Cool

BEAUTY BONUSES: Distinct cheekbones, well-shaped lips

AREAS TO TROUBLESHOOT: Uneven brows, wide nose

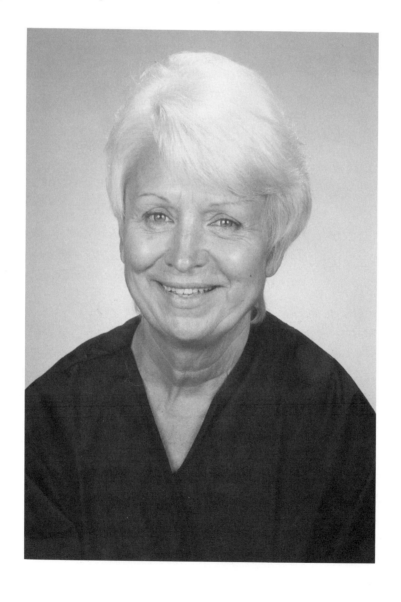

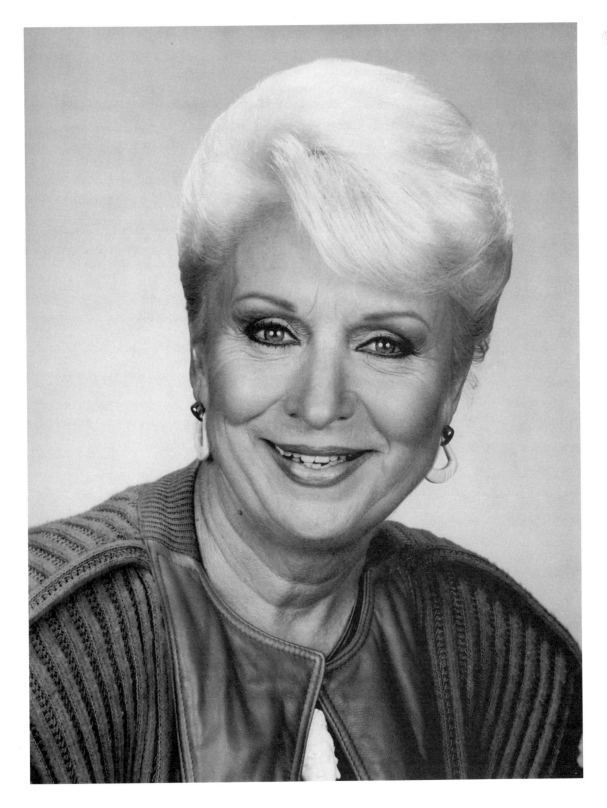

MARTHA GRESHAM'S MAKEOVER

There is no point in tampering with what is perfect to start with, and we all thought that Martha wears her hair just right. I simply gave it a little more finish—directing the side hair back and smoothing out the top.

I advised Martha against using heat appliances on her fine hair, such as hot rollers or curling irons. Her hair dries quickly, and she can style it with a blow dryer on a low setting. For someone with hair like hers, firm-hold styling mousse is a blessing. An egg-sized dollop combed through while the hair is damp gives it body and styleability.

We used porcelain concealer to cover her brown spots, and a fair foundation the same color as her skin. We dusted with loose powder.

Because she has distinct cheeks, we did not use contour on them, just a light watermelon blush on the bone line.

Martha's nose is very slightly bulbous at the tip, so we shaded the sides of her nose with taupe contour powder at the bottom to slim it down.

We needed to do some corrective work on her eyebrows, as the right one was curved and the left one was straight. We penciled in elegant arches on both sides, using taupe and mushroom pencils blended together with an eyebrow brush.

Martha has heavily lidded eyes. To counteract that, we applied oyster highlighter to her brow bones and extravagantly shaded and lined her lids in shades of gray.

Her well-shaped lips just needed some rose-pink lipstick.

As a businesswoman, Martha wants a look of "power". She's elegant and authoritative in her blue, leather-trimmed knit suit and distinctive ivory earrings and pendant.

ANGELA HYNES

"As one of the authors of this book and someone who has been silver since her early 20s, I staked my claim to be included in the makeovers.

"The original color of my hair was 'mousy'—a dull, medium brown with almost no highlights. Furthermore, it is fine and limp, with a couple of cowlicks that make it impossible to style. My hair really had nothing going for it. I was quite delighted when the silver started to grow in and give it some character. First I had silver streaks over each ear, then one above my left eye. Now that I'm thirty eight, it is almost totally white.

"My hair has gone from being my worst feature to one of my best. The color is a talking point. Strangers are always stopping me in the market or on the street to ask me about it! As I have fair skin and light gray eyes, the silver hair seems to suit me better than my original brown.

"I always wanted a long, flowing mane of hair, but mine is just too fine to look good that way. In any event, since I'm a certified workaholic and an exercise fanatic, it would be impractical to wear it long—I don't have the time or the inclination to take care of it. Instead, I keep it short on top so I can get some height, and always have hair at the nape of my neck for an illusion of length.

"My skin is the dry, fair, fine-textured type that is most susceptible to aging. I'm lucky that during my teens and twenties I lived in England, where the damp climate is particularly kind to skin. Now, however, I live at the beach in California. While researching this book, I scared myself half to death when I found out just how damaging the sun can be. I have vowed never to sunbathe again. It's doubtful I will keep that vow any longer than next summer, but at least I will never go out without sunblock on my face.

"If there were anything I could change about myself, I would wish to be taller. At five foot one, I have lived my life with the vague fear that I am being overlooked. I never can buy pants and skirts that don't have to be altered, and I've suffered from aching feet for years as a result of wearing high heels.

"The other drawback to being short is that a pound of fat that is unnoticable when distributed on a bigger person sits on me in a big lump. Although I eat sensibly, if I let up on exercising just a minute, fat globules invade my body from every direction. I try to keep them under control with a regular program of aerobics and yoga, both of which I enjoy enormously. It's my belief that physical activity is the key to maintaining a youthful outlook and appearance.

"Speaking of appearance, when it came to my turn for a makeover, I shamelessly asked my coauthor, Tony Ray, and the fantastic team of beauty experts at La Costa for a sexy look. Well, why not?"

ANGELA HYNES

HAIR ANALYSIS
Texture: Straight and very fine, however, it grows thickly on her scalp
Condition: Dry, with remnants of perm in longer hair at the nape
Percentage of Silver: Eighty on sides, fifty on top and at the back

FACE ANALYSIS
Skin Condition: Good, although tending to dryness; fine pores
Wrinkles: Crepiness around the eyes
Sun Damage: Minimal; a few freckles

COLOR PALETTE: True cool, with no yellow or red undertones

BEAUTY BONUSES: Well-shaped eyes and lips

AREAS TO TROUBLESHOOT: Hard-to-style hair, round face

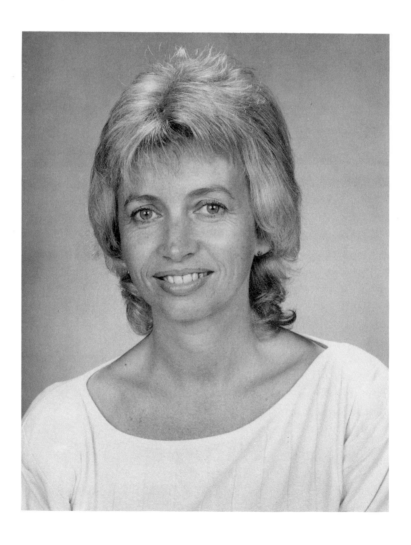

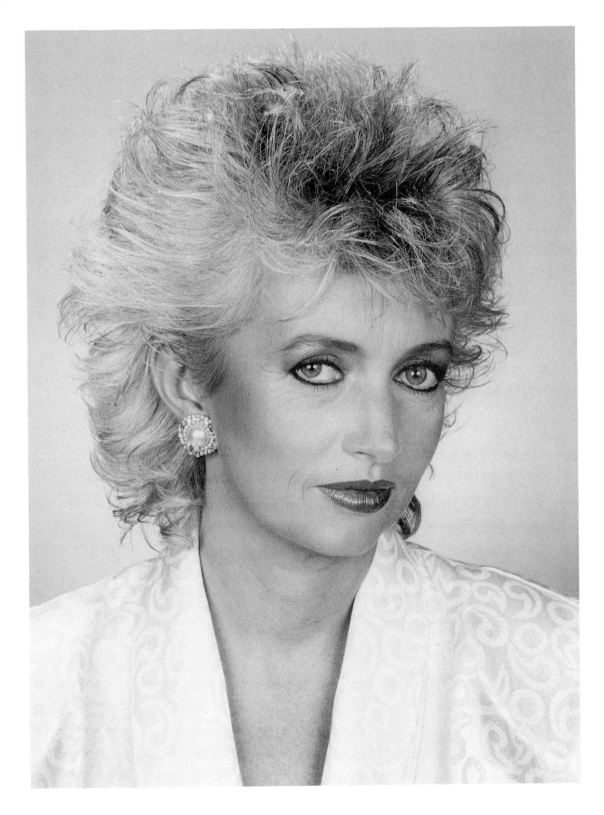

197

ANGELA HYNES'S MAKEOVER

Angela's hair was too fine and limp to take a cream rinse, but because it had a tendancy to be dry, I recommend she use a deep conditioner at home twice a month.

I didn't need to cut her hair, as the basic shape was good, though it was unimaginatively styled. I combed a good dollop of extrahold styling mousse through her wet hair to give it some volume.

It was rough-dried with a blow-dryer and finger-raked into shape. After back-combing the roots, I did the final styling with Paul Mitchell fast-drying sculpting hair spray—ideal for hard-to-style hair. By sweeping her hair back off her face at the sides, I reduced the width of her face and brought out her cheekbones. The "exploded" crown adds length to her height, and the tousled bangs give the casual, sexy look she wanted. With her hair fluffed up this way, more of her original brown color is visible, giving her hair a thicker, more textured look.

When it came to her face, I stressed the importance of using sunblock, moisturizer, and a good eye cream every single day. We smoothed on a moisture lotion and let it dry for a few minutes before starting to put on her makeup.

Angela's face was evened out with foundation in porcelain—the lightest "cool" color. Because her skin is dry, we did not use loose powder.

To give her a more defined chin, we blended a taupe contour powder from ear to ear just under her jawline and very carefully faded it into her neck.

Then we sculpted her cheeks with the same taupe contour powder applied under the bone, and a pink, slightly iridescent blush on the bone. Both were blended together. We applied highlighter to the center of her face from hairline to chin to give it length and make it look less full.

When it came to her eyes, we broke all the rules. Usually, I would not recommend dark charcoal eye liner for someone with such a fair complexion. But there were a couple of reasons for doing this. First, it helped draw attention away from the wrinkles around her eyes. Second, her irises are an extraordinarily light gray, and I decided to feature her eyes by contrasting them with dark eye makeup—the drama of the unexpected.

To balance the strong eyes, we used a deep-toned, muted-red lipstick. Her upper lip was uneven—thicker at one side than the other. We drew it in more symmetrically with lip pencil, and since she has a full lower lip, made that narrower by drawing just inside the natural line.

Angela is typical of fair-skinned women whose silver hair gives them a soft, luminous quality. In keeping with that, she wore a white-on-white silk jacket and large faux-pearl earrings. The chunky earrings draw attention to her sculpted cheekbones. The deep neck of the jacket adds length to her round face.

Did she get the sexy look she asked for? You be the judge.

JUDITH ANGEL

Raising six children kept Judith busy for years ("following them around is the best exercise in the world"), but when her youngest turned twelve, she decided to make a major adjustment and enter the work force. Now that she is forty-five, and the group coordinator of reservations at a hotel, her concern about her appearance and her awareness of herself are at an all-time high. "Looking good gives a person more confidence," she says. "If you really want something, you have to feel that you can go after it and get it!"

Despite the rigors of raising a big family, Judith has always taken some time for herself. She watches her diet carefully: At one point, she shed thirty pounds, which she's kept off ever since. "I don't deprive myself," she says. "I eat what I want, but I'm cautious about the size of the portions. I don't eat red meat, though. It isn't good for you, and all you miss is the chewing!" Judith also recommends getting plenty of sleep. "I get at least eight hours a night. I think that's incredibly important."

Her full-time job has limited her former bike-riding escapades (a twenty- or thirty-mile trip several times a week was de rigueur), and she confines her socializing to evenings at home with good friends.

Silver-haired since she was twenty, Judith firmly believes in sticking to what you have. "What would I possibly change it to?" she asks. "I get so many compliments on it! Some people even think I have it done this way. The silver is *me*. When the time came to decide what to do about my color, five out of my six kids said, 'Go for the silver!'" In fact, her twenty-three-year-old son already had silver growing in, and is happy to keep it that way too.

JUDITH ANGEL

HAIR ANALYSIS
Texture: Thick and curly
Condition: Dry from overperming
Percentage of Silver: Fifty

FACE ANALYSIS
Skin Condition: Normal
Wrinkles: Smile lines around her eyes
Sun Damage: Even suntan

COLOR PALETTE: Warm, with definite yellow undertones

BEAUTY BONUSES: Beautiful eyes and dazzling smile

AREAS TO TROUBLESHOOT: Sallow skin, dark undereye circles

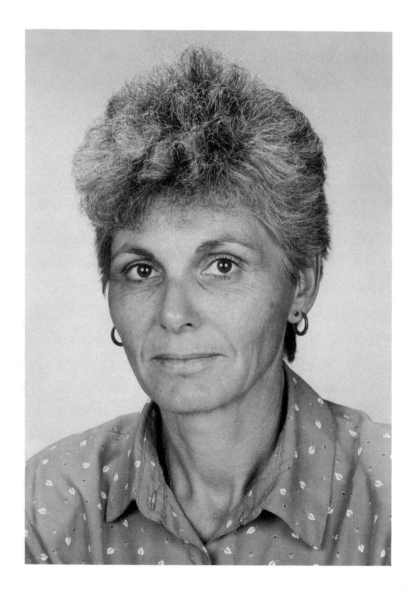

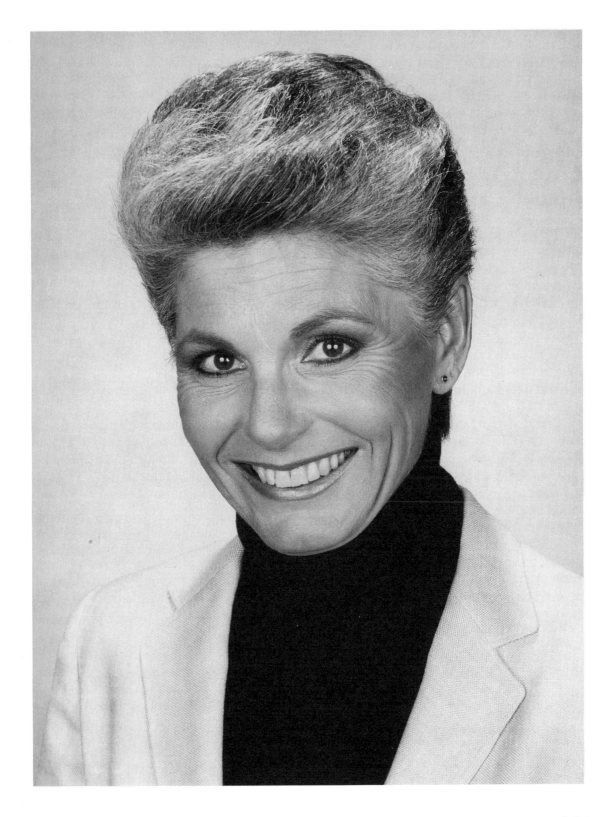

JUDITH ANGEL'S MAKEOVER

Judith is typical of those women whose salt and pepper hair looks wiry and coarse because it is curly. It was, in fact, dried out from over-processing, but was easily salvageable with a little know-how. The short, "boy" cut was good for her, but it needed smoothing into a straighter style that was not only much more chic, but also showed off the growth pattern of the gray and gave the impression that her hair was healthy and shiny.

I gave it a deep conditioning and recommended that she do the same every month.

Then I simply blow dried it back off her face in a modern version of a pompadour. Because her hair is thick, it could take a dab of styling glaze, which I rubbed between my palms and slicked over her hair to keep it in place. What a difference in her appearance already!

Judith has an olive complexion. She needed makeup colors from the pinker end of the warm spectrum of colors to give her a glow. We used a rose-tan concealer on the dark circles under her eyes, around her lips, and on the bridge of her sun-tanned nose before blending on rachel foundation.

As we did not use powder, we highlighted her cheeks with a cream rather than a powder blush. Three dots of peach-colored blush were dabbed along her cheekbone and blended with the fingertips up toward her temples.

We tidied up her brows by tweezing a little from the *inside*, and giving more definition with a sable pencil to the natural line on the *outside*.

Judith has beautiful brown eyes that deserved special emphasis. We used peach blush instead of eye shadow as a base and highlighter on her lid. Contour eye shadow in the crease was soft copper and we accented that with a wedge of teal blue, blended up and out, at the outer corners. Smudged liner and mascara were both soft brown.

Like her eyes, her big smile was emphasized. We outlined her lips with a coral pencil and filled in with brick lipstick. Her lips were a little dry, so we gave them some softness with a slick of clear gloss.

Judith is breaking all the color rules—and looks smashing in the process! It just goes to show that, although we've offered you sound guidelines, ultimately you must go by what looks good on *you*. Normally, someone with sallow skin should not wear black next to her face. However, we warmed up her complexion with peaches and corals, and as she still has a good deal of dark color in her hair, the black works. It's tempered, too, by the white jacket.

A look this clean-cut needs no jewelry. The result? Chic, sophisticated, and very classy.

MARY RYMAN

Mary, forty-nine, and her husband love fishing, but that's not nearly as sedentary as it sounds. They take off for Minnesota or Canada and trek for miles to their favorite spots (sorry, but she won't disclose any secret locales). "We usually camp out," she says. "Nothing is as good for you as all that fresh air and exercise."

She balances her outdoor exploits with a fondness for dancing at a club she belongs to. She'd far rather have dinner out with friends and spend the night burning up the dance floor than entertain at home.

Despite her well-balanced social life, Mary feels she doesn't spend as much time on herself as she should. "I don't have lots of time for salons and appointments. I look the best I can without dwelling on it. Besides, I think *attitude* is the most important beauty asset. How you're feeling shows on your face and can really affect your looks."

Her best trait? According to her, a warm smile that comes from a positive attitude. If she could change anything about herself, it would be her tendency to procrastinate about exercise. "I'm the worst! I rationalize that I'm too busy and will do it later. Consequently, I don't exercise as much as I should."

Mary also exemplifies a certain adaptability. Part of that stems from working as an executive secretary on and off for thirty years and raising four sons in between. "Letting go of them was the hardest thing I ever did," she says. "They were close in age, so when they started to leave home, they all seemed to go at once. It was traumatic, because we also moved from Illinois at the same time. Actually, going through so much turned out to be good for my marriage."

Change has been a byword when it comes to her appearance, too. "I've colored my hair from time to time, but now I'm thinking of not doing it any more. The silver softens everything as you get older. Why battle something that's obviously a grand plan?"

MARY RYMAN

HAIR ANALYSIS
Texture: Fine
Condition: Permed
Percentage of Silver: Sixty

FACE ANALYSIS
Skin Condition: Normal to dry
Wrinkles: Primarily around the lips
Sun Damage: Very little; some brown spots

COLOR PALETTE: Cool

BEAUTY BONUSES: Warm smile, attractive silvering in her hair

AREA TO TROUBLESHOOT: Double chin

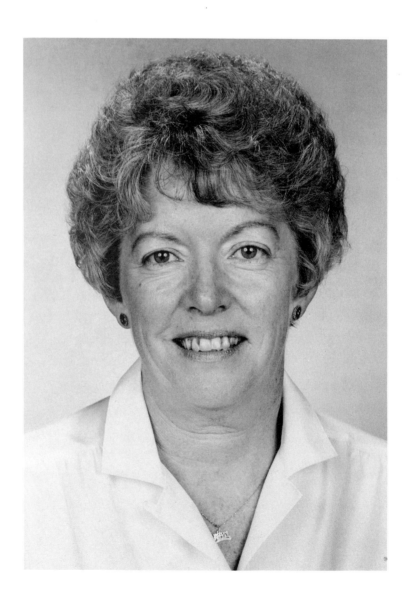

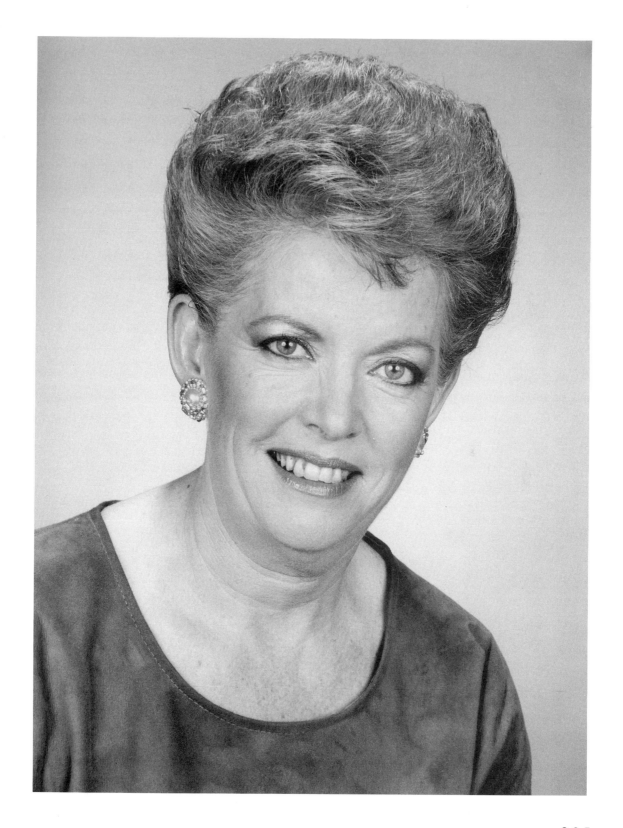

MARY RYMAN'S MAKEOVER

Mary is one of those women whose hair has gone gray evenly throughout—there are no defined streaks. The effect, therefore, is very soft. Because her hair is finely textured, she perms it for body. A good idea, but I felt that the style was, frankly, dull. She needed a more up-to-date look. I trimmed the sides and back, but left the top longer. Her sleeker style was achieved by directing her hair back and up, over a small, round styling brush. The perm helped me achieve fullness on top. The upswept sides gave her whole face a lift.

A little rose concealer on Mary's nose and brown patches evened out her skin tone before we dabbed on and blended in rose-beige foundation and fluffed on loose powder.

Her full face needed some contouring, so we shaded around her hairline from temples to mouth level with taupe powder.

We used the same taupe to deal with her double chin. It was brushed on just under the jawline and down her throat a little. We blended a little highlighter on the center of her chin to make it more defined.

Mary is a good example of someone whose features were beautifully enhanced by the clever use of color. The intense concentration of blue and gray eye shadows and charcoal eyeliner make her gray eyes look lighter—more sparkly—and the whites clearer. It's noticeable even in these black-and-white photographs.

Similarly, her smile—which she regards as her best feature—is much brighter when her teeth are made to look whiter, by contrasting them with the blue-red fuchsia lipstick we applied.

Her lips, incidentally, were dry and cracked. Before brushing on lip color, we conditioned them with a moisturizing lip fixative that also helps stop color from feathering into the tiny lines around her mouth.

Mary's overall look is soft and muted. We kept it that way by dressing her in a soft, gunmetal-gray suede top that beautifully complemented her hair.

LOUISE CABRAL

Versatility and a passion for the arts fill Louise's days. She has retired from full-time duties teaching English and drama but is still "addicted" to teaching and enjoys part-time work at a school in Agoura, California. Her love of acting and writing have prompted her to develop a course for senior citizens called "That Book You Always Wanted To Write," in which students are encouraged to write their autobiographies—not for publication, but as a legacy for their families.

Louise, who is "in her fifties," cites a terrible bout of writer's block that lasted for weeks as one of the turning points of her life. "I thought I'd go mad!" she says. A lesson emerged: the necessity for self-discipline. She plants herself at her desk at 5:30 A.M. every day and proceeds to write *all* morning. "That's because life is my religion, and writing is my way of praying."

She confines most of her socializing to dancing, particularly when her artist husband accompanies her to the clubs where her daughter sings. Her other child is a former flamenco guitarist turned social worker.

Her advice to women? "Keep a journal, and write in it every day. It sounds corny, but it helps you find yourself. When you have to make decisions, it helps to put your true thoughts and feelings on paper." She is also very goal-oriented. "Goals are important—even if you never reach them!"

Louise takes a similarly exuberant and matter-of-fact view of herself. "I like lots of makeup," she asserts. "I refuse to look 'old.' And when I decide that I need a plastic surgeon, I'll go to one."

LOUISE CABRAL

HAIR ANALYSIS
Texture: Thick, straight
Condition: Good
Percentage of Silver: One hundred

FACE ANALYSIS
Skin Condition: Dry
Wrinkles: Some around the eyes
Sun Damage: Isolated brown spots

COLOR PALETTE: Warm

BEAUTY BONUS: Classic oval face

AREAS TO TROUBLESHOOT: Overtweezed eyebrows

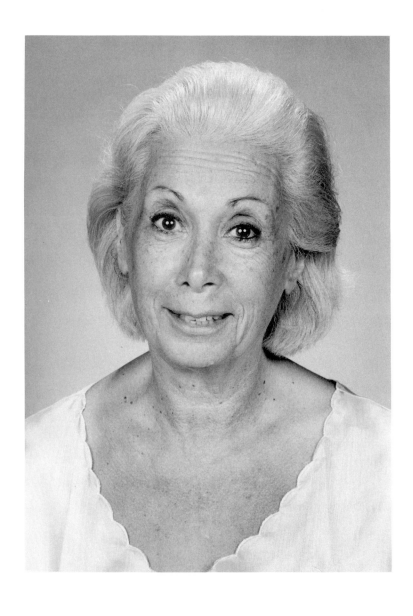

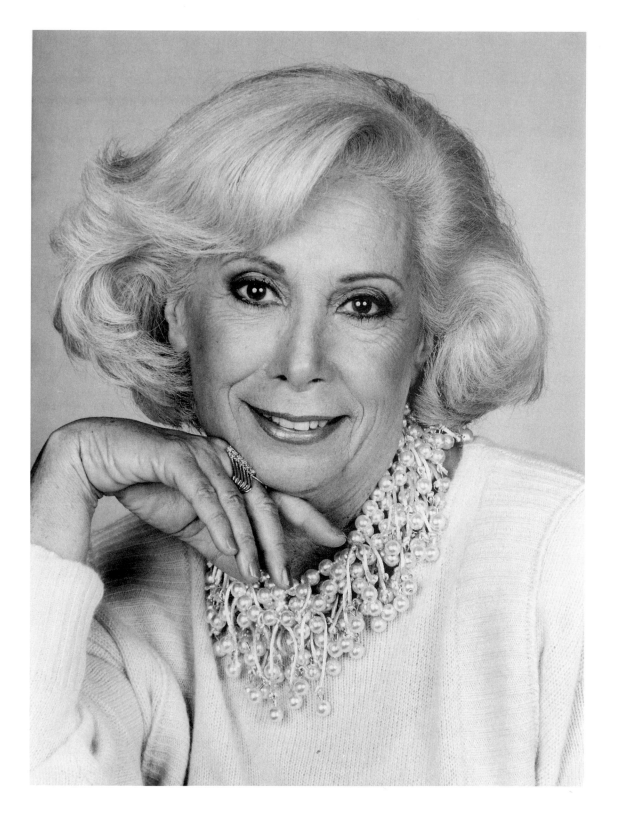

LOUISE CABRAL'S MAKEOVER

Louise's original hair color was very dark. She has lost her brown and red tones but still has a touch of yellow, giving her hair a beautiful pale platinum appearance rather than true silver. Her swept-back style—while showing off the color—was a little too severe. I cut in some long bangs to soften her high forehead.

Then I set her hair on large sponge curlers, with the bangs to the side, the top straight back, and the sides down. When loosely combed out, her hair fell in an easy, unstudied style, with width at the sides, which accentuated her cheeks.

Louise is very lucky to have a face that needs no contouring. A little ivory concealer took care of the brown spots, and a honey-beige foundation and translucent powder fluffed onto her face gave her a glowing complexion.

We simply added a little peach blush stroked directly on her cheekbones and blended up toward her temples.

Louise had overtweezed her brows (a common problem with many of our makeover subjects). We corrected them by drawing in feathery strokes with light- and medium-brown pencils. We used peach blush on her lids as a base for a mellow ginger contour shadow and sable-brown eye liner and mascara.

We created fuller, wider lips by lining with coral pencil on the outer edge of her natural line and then smudging it so the line blended naturally into the same-colored lipstick. A slick of peach gloss on her lips completed the picture.

A buttercream sweater and a cascade of peachy pearls is soft and feminine. In fact, it's all peaches and cream!

CHARLENE BASKIN

Charlene is always on the run. Whether it's after her two children, ages five and nine, or during her daily three-to-four-mile jog, she likes to stay constantly on the move. But she also remembers exactly where she's been. Although she made the leap from Minneapolis to the West Coast fifteen years ago, she cites good, solid Midwestern values as the creed she lives by.

Time spent with her children—in addition to the fact that she's approaching forty—has made her increasingly conscious about herself. "I'm more aware of a need for time all to myself," she says. "As your child's life is going on, so is yours. Your life is being spent as well."

Part of her formula for dealing with that is to enjoy the theater or dressing up for a fine restaurant. "My husband and I try to do that once a week," she says. "As a parent who spends so much of the week in sweats, I need it!"

Allowing personal time is coupled with a pride in herself as an individual. "That's what my silver hair gives me," says Charlene. "It's never occurred to me to color it; that would not be me! In any event, I don't have time for beauty shops." Charlene is the cousin of Carey Simon, one of our other models—it seems that beautiful silver hair runs in the family.

CHARLENE BASKIN

HAIR ANALYSIS
Texture: Thick, straight
Condition: Excellent
Percentage of Silver: Seventy-five

FACE ANALYSIS
Skin Condition: Normal
Wrinkles: Minimal; smile lines around the eyes
Sun Damage: Patchy tan

COLOR PALETTE: Warm

BEAUTY BONUSES: Beautiful teeth and smile

AREAS TO TROUBLESHOOT: Dowdy hairstyle, hooded eyes

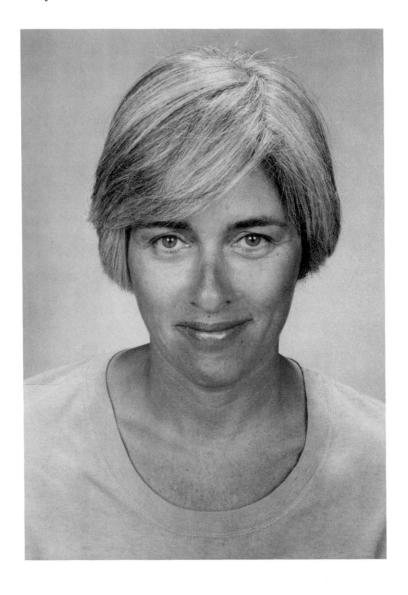

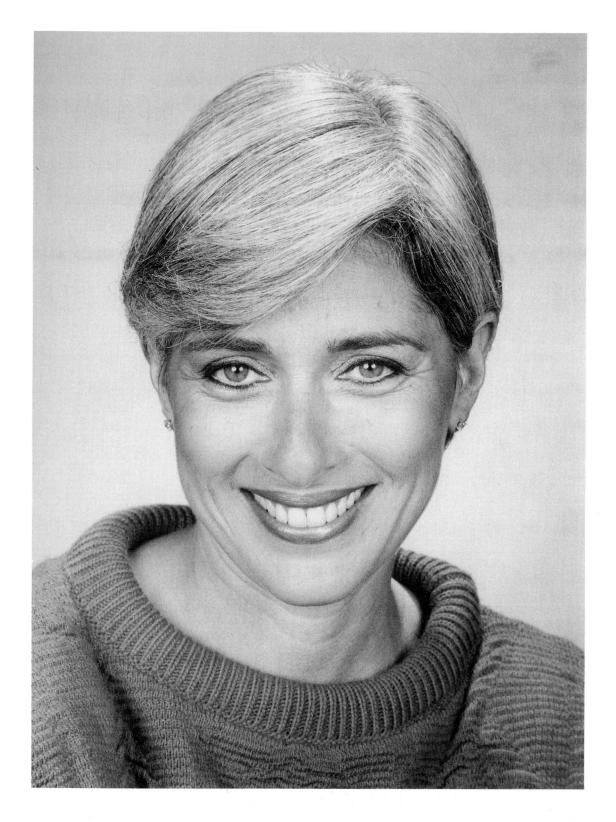

213

CHARLENE BASKIN'S MAKEOVER

Charlene is growing out a short style, so she didn't want me to cut her hair. The condition of her hair was good; all she needed was a cream rinse to give it shine. Her color is dramatic enough to be worn in a simple style, but I thought she would look fresher and more youthful if it were just tucked behind her ears. I was right! A light misting of hair spray kept it in place all day.

Charlene suffers from a classic Sunbelt condition—"sunglasses syndrome." She has pale circles around her eyes, while the rest of her face is tan. We evened out her face color with two tones of foundation—honey on the darker skin, and rachel around her eyes—carefully blended on her skin with a damp sea sponge.

To play up her cheeks, we swept salmon blush from the "apple" of her cheek up toward her hairline and added just a touch of creamy highlighter on top of that, on the fullest part of her cheekbones.

Charlene tends to have hooded lids, so we tweezed her heavy brows from the undersides to widen the space between lash and brow lines. We did not highlight her brow bone, as this tends to play up the problem. Instead, we applied rich copper shadow in her lid crease and faded it upward to diminish the overhang.

We painted on a very fine dark brown line on upper and lower lids. A flick of brown-black mascara completed her eye makeup.

A kiss of tomato-red lipstick on her lip line plays up her great smile.

Charlene's style is simple and charming. All she needed was a chic sweater in terra cotta, which complemented her sleek hairstyle and warm coloring.

MAGGI GLADDEN

She's retired now that she's seventy-two, but Maggi ("I don't feel comfortable with Margaret; I'm definitely a Maggi") possesses unflagging energy. She entered the business world after high school, and for forty-three years worked with her husband as an interior designer in a family-owned firm. They raised four children (and now have ten grandchildren and six great-grandchildren!). Maggi enjoys painting oil portraits and playing tennis several times a week. She recently took up tap dancing to improve her grace and movement on the court!

A Russian-born, former British subject, whose father worked in Russia and fled with his family during the Revolution, Maggi is not intimidated by travel or change. She's been to Turkey and Greece with her husband this year, and has plans to see the Great Barrier Reef next year.

Her social life ranges from extravagant club functions to quiet dinners at home with her husband ("He's great company!"). Whether she's out on the town or in the confines of her home, Maggi takes tremendous pride in her appearance. "I'm concerned about older women taking more care of themselves, as opposed to 'letting themselves go.' Staying slim is very important, and sometimes that means restraint! It's like a kid with candy. When you get old enough to buy all you want, you should know enough not to eat it. You can enjoy it *all*, but in moderation.

"Keep a healthy sense of competition as you grow older. It keeps you on your toes and prevents you from becoming smug. Competition should be your spark! After all, we're always competing for something."

Maggi also believes that mixing with younger people helps keep you youthful. "I feel I've held up my end. I've maintained my physical strength and can keep up with women half my age. That's not bragging; it's healthy."

MAGGI GLADDEN

HAIR ANALYSIS
Texture: Fine
Condition: Permed and slightly dry
Percentage of Silver: One hundred

FACE ANALYSIS
Skin Condition: Dry
Wrinkles: Around the eyes, mouth, and lips
Sun Damage: Freckles and brown patches

COLOR PALETTE: Cool

BEAUTY BONUSES: Irrepressible youthful sparkle

AREAS TO TROUBLESHOOT: Scar on right brow, slightly discolored teeth

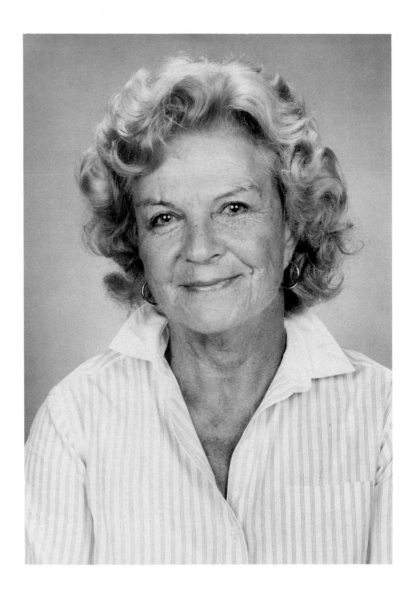

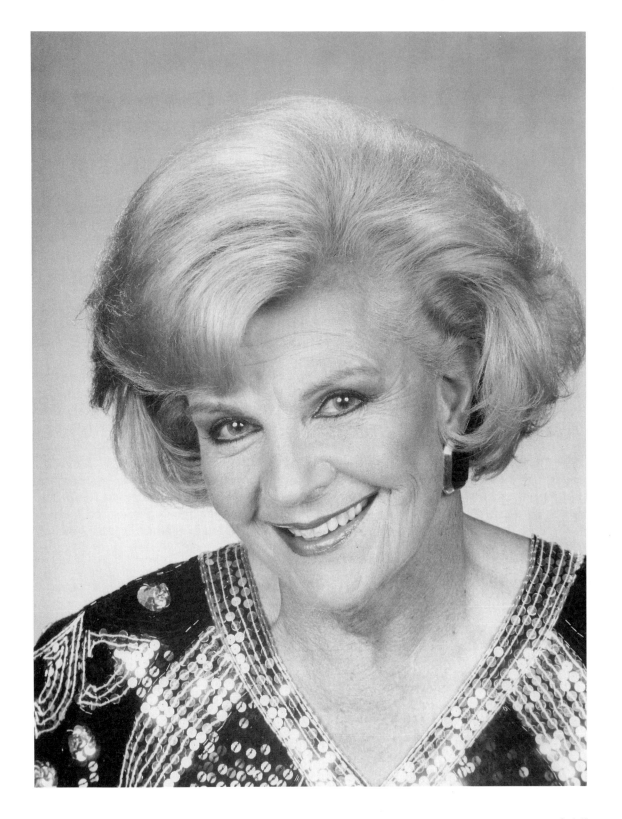

MAGGI GLADDEN'S MAKEOVER

I started out having a small argument with Maggi over her hair. I wanted to cut off some of the permed length and give her a straighter style, but she was resistant. After seeing how some of our other makeovers turned out, however, she decided to give me a chance.

I lopped an inch from the bottom and, after washing her hair, combed a setting lotion through it and set it in large rollers. The rollers were set back except for her bangs, which were rolled to the side.

Maggi sat under a hood dryer on medium heat for fifteen minutes and came out from under it while her hair was still very slightly damp. I removed the curlers and let her hair finish drying naturally. Then I brushed it out in the direction of the curl and back-combed it a little at the roots for fullness. Tucked behind her ears, this straighter, bobbed style framed her face beautifully. The deep, sideswept bangs helped cover the scar on her brow. Her fine hair needed a touch of firm-hold hair spray to keep it in style.

Maggi had a few brown patches, which we concealed before applying a rose-mist foundation and a well-buffed dusting of translucent powder. We not only used fuchsia blush directly on her cheekbones, but gave her whole face a glow by dusting it sparingly on her temples, chin, and between her brows.

We filled in her brows—including the scarred area—not with a pencil, but with a smoky-gray pressed-powder eyeshadow applied with a brush. It had a softening effect.

To counteract the effect of Maggi's widely spaced eyes, we took wine eye shadow well into the inner center of her lids and faded it toward the outer corners. Soft lilac highlighter on the brow bone and dark gray liner rimmed top and bottom lids enhanced the gray-blue color of her twinkling eyes.

We gave her upper lid a more defined cupid's bow with a blue-red pencil. Rich, glossy plum lipstick and a slick of gloss for after-dark sizzle completed the makeup. The blue-red color helped whiten and detract attention from her slightly discolored teeth.

Maggi's exotic black evening gown, softened with light reflecting sequins, and jet-and-silver earrings are simply stunning. Her whole look just *sparkles* with life and youth.

NICKI STINTON

Nicki, thirty-six, takes time out from her job as a graphic designer to play tennis and ski ("Taos, New Mexico, is probably my favorite place"), but yoga is the athletic mainstay she most enjoys. "I lift a few weights now and then, but I'm not an exercise fanatic," she explains.

"I try to make time for myself," she says. "It's refreshing to walk in the hills and have a few quiet, reflective moments."

Going to restaurants and movies gives Nicki a chance to socialize, and although she likes dressing up, she finds the "California casual" ambience doesn't provide as many suitable occasions as the theaters back home, in London. Often, she will prepare a casual dinner for four to six friends.

When we shot this photograph, Nicki was pregnant with her first child. Since then, she and her photographer husband have had a little boy—Halley (for the comet) Mark Twain (for her husband's hero) Stinton.

Nicki's hair began turning silver in her mid-twenties, and she discovered that blues and purples suited her new look perfectly. "I've gone through phases with tints and rinses, but I always go back to silver. I used to darken it in the summer, when I got tanned, but now I don't bother anymore. I get more compliments with it as it is, anyway. I wouldn't ever go back to some all-over flat color . . . silver highlights are great."

NICKI STINTON

HAIR ANALYSIS
Texture: Medium; grows densly
Condition: Normal, with dry, split ends
Percentage of Silver: Forty

FACE ANALYSIS
Skin Condition: Excellent
Wrinkles: Very few around the eyes, deep lines from nose to mouth
Sun Damage: Almost none; uneven tan

COLOR PALETTE: Warm

BEAUTY BONUS: Beautiful skin

AREAS TO TROUBLESHOOT: Wide face

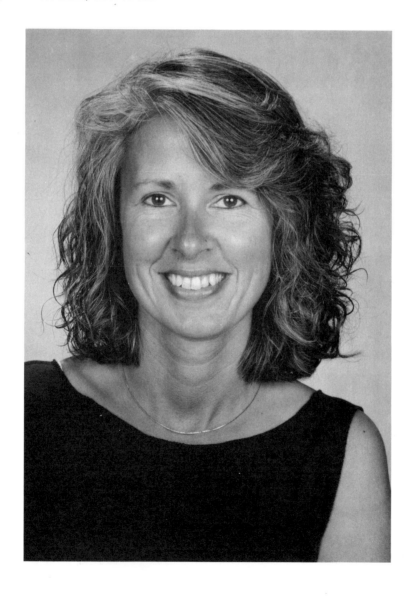

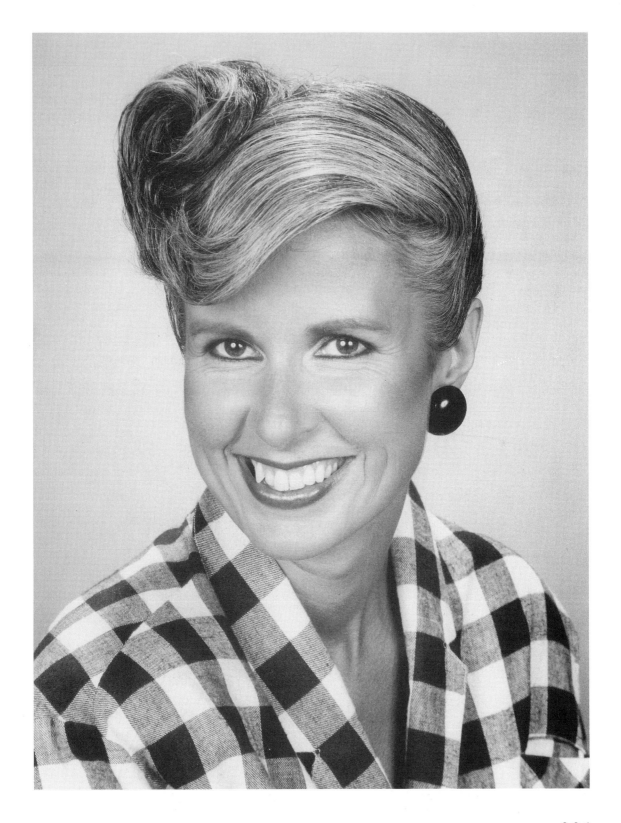

221

NICKI STINTON'S MAKEOVER

As an art director involved in the fashion world, Nicki sports a casual, trendy look. She wanted to keep her hair length, so I showed her how to achieve a slightly more sophisticated style without effecting any drastic changes. I just snipped off a few dry ends.

Her hair has a slightly yellow cast. After washing it, I combed through a bit of Fancifull's mousse in White Minx to hold the style while toning down the gold.

I blow dried her hair straight before folding it up into a classic French twist. The twist on this twist?—it's on the *side* instead of at the back! All her hair was brushed over to one side and held—like a ponytail—in one hand. Then I folded it over my hand to form a smooth twist.

Nicki's glowing complexion (remember, she was pregnant!) needed only minimum coverage. We used no concealer, just slicked on a fine layer of ivory foundation to even out her skin tone, and left off both powder and blush for a natural look.

We did, however, use mocha contour powder to slim down her wide, angular face a little. We blended it at the outside corners of her temples and jawline.

Her deeply set eyes were most enhanced with just a sweep of light turquoise over the entire lid and gently smudged eye liner in deep olive on the top and bottom lids. Brown mascara completed the picture.

Nicki's huge, warm smile sparkled with perssimon lipstick and a slick of clear gloss.

A big-shouldered white-and-olive jacket and simple olive earrings completed a fresh, crisp, professional look.

PHYLLIS FIRTEL

Phyllis, sixty-four, never misses a daily workout in her backyard pool. "I swim as long as I can last," she says with a laugh. "It's different every time." Out on terra firma, she's an avid reader, with a special weakness for a good mystery. She also relaxes by knitting clothing for her granddaughter.

She and her husband are theater aficionados, but Phyllis makes certain that the two of them have plenty of time together at home. "We like both formal and casual evenings," she explains.

What keeps her going is a nonanxious view of life. "You should enjoy yourself, and not worry about every little thing," she advises. "Finding time for your loved ones is the most important of all. I'm better now at living with the bumps in life than I was, but it takes work."

Phyllis takes a similar no-fuss-and-bother tack when it comes to plastic surgery. "I don't believe in it for cosmetic reasons," she says. "If I really needed it for my health, that would be different."

She treats her silver hair with the same sensible, highly personal code. "It began turning white in my twenties. It came in slowly, and the white strands contrasting with the dark were very striking. I've always loved it. I don't want to be a slave to the beauty parlor, but I thought perhaps my family would like me to look younger, so I offered to color my hair. They said, 'Absolutely not.' "

PHYLLIS FIRTEL

HAIR ANALYSIS
Texture: Thick and strong
Condition: Healthy
Percentage of Silver: Ninety

FACE ANALYSIS
Skin Condition: Dry and coarsely textured
Wrinkles: Extensive
Sun Damage: Extensive

COLOR PALETTE: Warm

BEAUTY BONUSES: Excellent hair; well-shaped lips

AREA TO TROUBLESHOOT: Abused skin

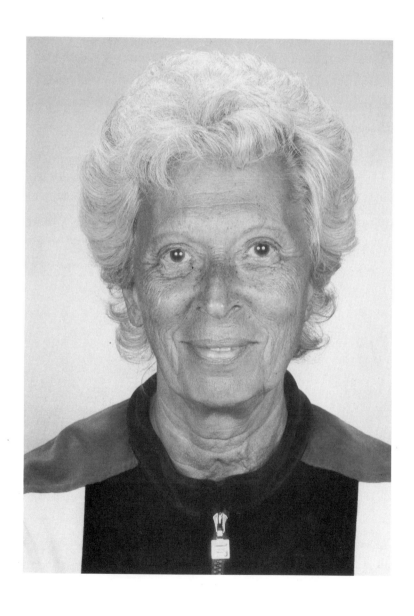

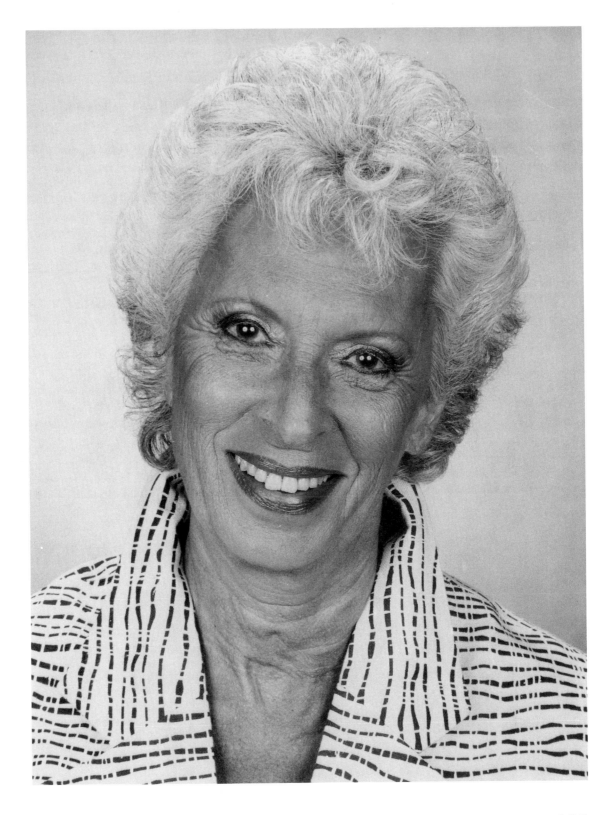

PHYLLIS FIRTEL'S MAKEOVER

Why try to improve on perfection? Phyllis's silver hair is strong, healthy, and shiny. Her softly tousled style suited her perfectly. I simply trimmed a millimeter off the ends to eradicate some dryness. Then I washed it, towel-dried it, and let it dry naturally into its usual shape.

I recommended that she use hair-care products that have a sunscreen in order to maintain her good hair condition.

Phyllis really needed assistance with her facial skin. She is guilty of inflicting considerable sun damage on her skin, and before we did anything else, we applied moisturizer to smooth out the rough, dry surface.

We chose not to use a concealer, since it would have looked too artificial against her very tanned skin. Instead, we applied a couple of layers of tan foundation with a very damp sponge. That effectively evened out the color. We passed on powder (it would have settled in her lines and looked caked).

Because Phyllis has an oval face and good cheekbones, blush was kept subtle. Peach powder blush was fluffed on her cheekbones and extended up to her temples.

We very lightly penciled in brows with a muted brown pencil. Rather than using a dark eye shadow in the socket, we used a pale salmon over her entire lid, and an accent color of earthy green swept up at the outer corners. Raisin-brown eye liner was smudged and blended into the shadow for a soft look. We used dark brown on top and bottom lids.

Phyllis's lips are full, with a good cupid's bow. Her top lip is slightly uneven, but it gives her an individualistic smile. So we outlined her lips and used a bright coral lipstick to show off her dazzlingly white teeth and bright smile.

Phyllis keeps her outdoorsy look in a sporty black-and-white jacket. The V neck and turned up collar draw attention away from her rather lined throat. The effect is crisp, contemporary, and very flattering.

CHARLENE ARRINGTON

After working as an executive secretary for thirty-five years, Charlene, fifty-five, now works for her husband in the petroleum-marketing field. Since they're fresh-air/sports-minded people, they balance their office work with walking, golf, and a La Costa-inspired routine that includes the rebounder, walking, a rowing machine, and a sauna.

"Exercise is one of the pleasures of living in California," says Charlene, who is adamant about making time for a workout at least three times a week. "In fact, we make a habit of not going out often in order to fit sleep into our health program! I believe in a simple life-style, and feel that if you're physically fit, you're happier and can accomplish more. What you are on the inside is reflected on the outside."

She's had to battle a tendency toward perfectionism along the way. "I've learned that no matter how fast you try to go, outside influences will slow you down. That teaches you patience." It has also taught her that reaching for happiness is of paramount importance. "It isn't difficult if you always look on the bright side. Greet each new day . . . laugh about it . . . face it . . . and get on with living."

Charlene's hair showed its first hint of silver when she was eighteen, and by the time she was twenty-eight, the process was complete. "I colored it then, but I haven't since I was forty," she says. "I don't think that's good for it, and I want to keep my hair healthy. I'm eternally grateful for it now. My grandchildren look at me and think I'm an angel!"

CHARLENE ARRINGTON

HAIR ANALYSIS
Texture: Thick, with a natural wave
Condition: Good; healthy
Percentage of Silver: Ninety

FACE ANALYSIS
Skin condition: Normal; enlarged pores
Wrinkles: Crepey around the eyes, deep creases from nose to mouth
Sun Damage: Brown spots around eyes and on forehead

COLOR PALETTE: Cool

BEAUTY BONUS: Healthy hair

AREAS TO TROUBLESHOOT: Drooping eyes; jowly jawline

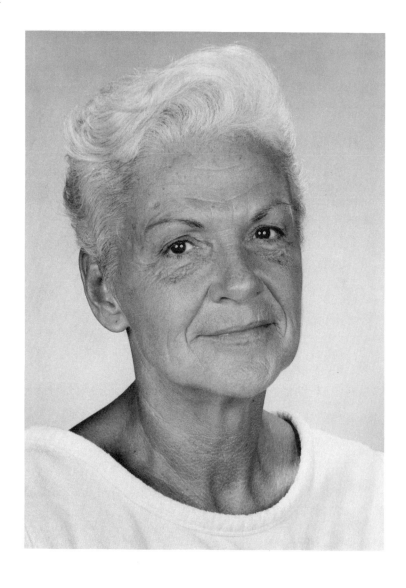

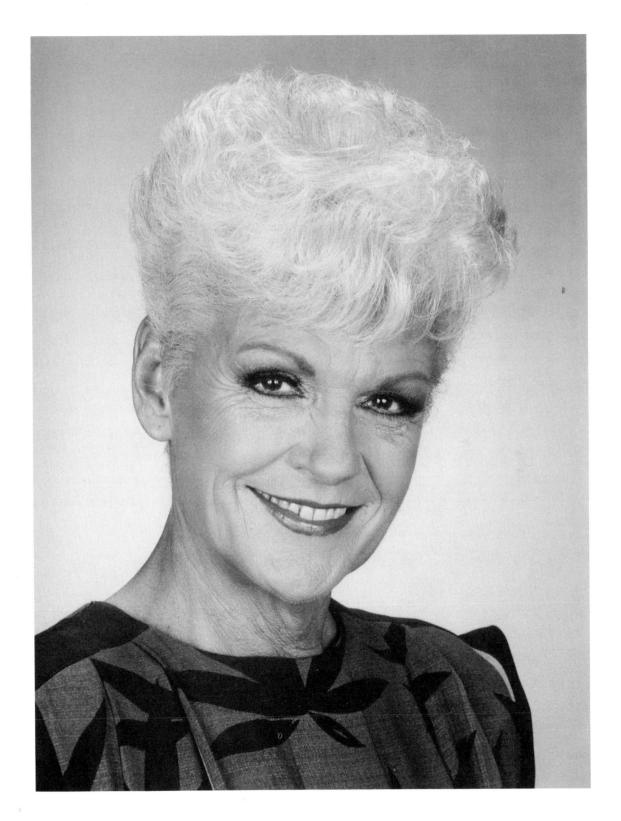

CHARLENE ARRINGTON'S MAKEOVER

Charlene just needed to add spark to a simple style. By directing the hair on her crown forward, instead of back, she gets a softer, more face-framing look. Her naturally wavy hair is easy to style. After blow drying her hair, I used a curling iron on top (just for a few seconds), and did a little back-combing at the roots, to get a looser effect.

I slicked the sides straight back, and held it all in place with a spritz of light-hold hair spray.

Charlene tends to have dark circles under her eyes. We countered that with carefully blended rose-tan concealer, and also applied concealer in the lines between nose and mouth.

We broke the rules about not trying to change the color of your skin with foundation and applied a color one shade lighter than her face. This was because her extremely tanned skin contrasted rather startlingly with her pale hair. This needs to be done with care, and we *meticulously* blended around her jawline. We did not use powder.

We applied taupe contour around her jawline from ear to ear to diminish the width of her jowls.

To slim her face even further, we blended a little highlighter down the center of her face—between the brows and down the nose and the center of her chin.

Her cheeks got a light blush of pink on the bone.

Charlene's brows were well shaped but thin. We supplemented them with taupe and light gray pencil lines.

Her eyes tend to droop at the outer corners. After shading them with a soft-pink highlighter and eggplant contour swept upward, we gave her eyes an appealing lift with false lashes. In this case, we applied charcoal-gray strip—as opposed to individual— "glamour" lashes: thick, and varying in length. The effect? Bold, but not brazen.

Strong, clear red lip pencil and lipstick provide a counterpoint to her newly defined eyes.

A print dress in shades of taupe, wine, and purple further brightens Charlene's complexion, and the overall look is contemporary and energetic.

JANE KUGELMAN

Jane, fifty-seven, keeps active with charity work in her community and develops her energy by exercising religiously. She'll walk up to twenty miles per day or use a La Costa trampoline when it's raining too hard to go outdoors. "If I don't make time to exercise, I'm lethargic all day," she says. She also recommends fresh air, no smoking, and only moderate drinking to increase stamina. "All that walking also gives you time to think things through, and that's as important as the exercise."

When she's up and about, though, Jane does everything in a big way. She considers a small dinner party to be twelve people, and a small cocktail party to be about a hundred. She's a voracious traveler as well; Canada is a particular favorite. "Leave those furs and bulky coats at home,"she advises. "Travel light. A good Burberry trenchcoat with a zip-out lining is invaluable, and a strand of pearls works wonders with everything."

Jane hardly looks like a woman old enough to have four daughters and seven grandchildren, but she attributes much of her happiness to her belief in "staying young."

"Don't be selfish, but go ahead and think about yourself: your body . . . your looks . . . your health. Those things are important to your husband and children too!"

Her hair turned silver when she hit thirty. "Everybody likes it, and I'm comfortable with it. I love to wear white, black, and red! As for 'character lines.' I think they're part of a woman's beauty. If you have good skin, leave yourself alone!"

JANE KUGELMAN

HAIR ANALYSIS
Texture: Thick, straight, and wiry
Condition: Dry
Percentage of Silver: Fifty

FACE ANALYSIS
Skin Condition: Oily, with enlarged pores
Wrinkles: Some around eyes; deep creases between nose and mouth
Sun Damage: Minimal

COLOR PALETTE: Warm

BEAUTY BONUSES: Beautiful eyes

AREAS TO TROUBLESHOOT: "Flat" face, with little definition

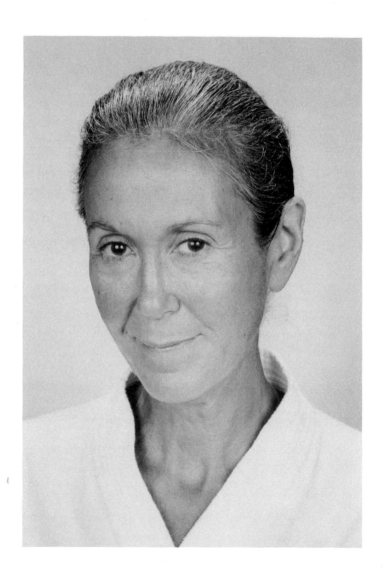

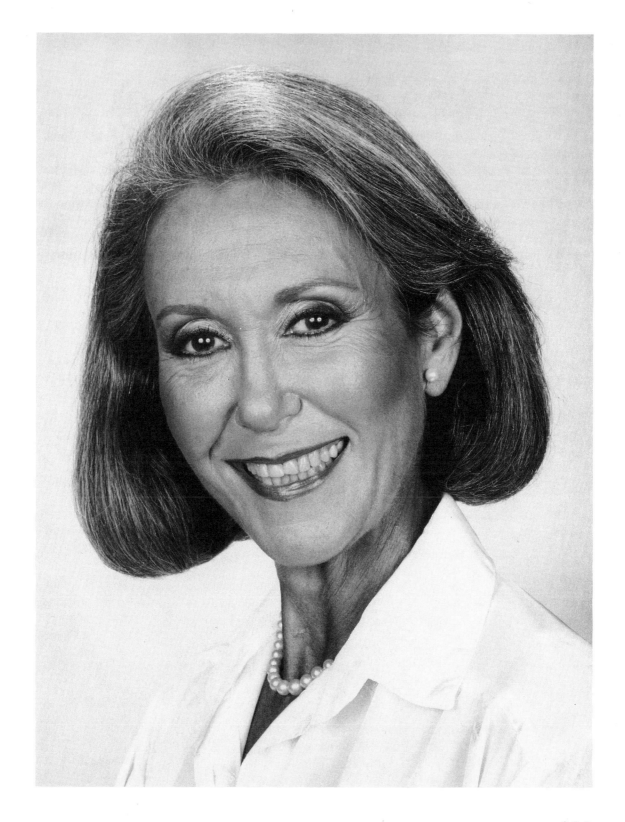

233

JANE KUGELMAN'S MAKEOVER

Jane had been controlling her wiry, iron-gray, hair by pulling it straight back. I let it loose! I snipped a little off the bottom, and, after giving it a conditioning to add shine to her dry hair, blow dried it into a polished bob. This sideswept top is universally flattering, and the length balances her narrow chin. This is how coarse, thick hair can be made to look soft and sexy.

Jane is a sun worshipper—but fortunately, her skin is quite oily so it has not become too dehydrated. Rose-tan concealer was blended in the lines between nose and mouth, and a tan foundation gives her skin an even finish. A well-buffed dusting of loose powder helps stop the shine.

Jane's face is somewhat "flat." We created depth by contouring under her cheekbone and up toward her temples with sienna, then highlighting on the bone with a lighter, peachy blush.

Highlighter at the outside edge of her forehead and along the top edge of her jawline helped balance her diamond-shaped face.

It was easy to add drama to her beautiful eyes by applying a soft peach shadow on the brow bone, brushing burnished copper in the socket, and lining the top and bottom with dark brown liner. Dark brown mascara adds the final touch.

Lip color in persimmon accents her mouth and balances her eyes.

Cream silk and pearls—what more needs to be said? What could look more classy?

PENNY McGARRY

You've seen Penny as our model throughout this book. Now take a look at her before-and-after transformation! At twenty-eight, she's the youngest of our makeovers. Like some of our other models, she's decided to live with and enjoy her prematurely silver hair.

Penny's a native of England, but enjoys the United States (where she works as a retail representative), and plans to stay here. The California life-style suits her gregarious nature. She loves tennis and swimming, but prefers not to be too regimented about working out. She's active and outgoing—especially when it comes to cocktail parties or the movies ("I love Spielberg films!")

"People like my hair short like this," she says. "I usually wear it in a softly curled style, but when I'm going out on the town—something special, such as dancing at a club—I do spike it up a bit." She also does special things with her makeup to complement her hair. "I like muted tones. I don't wear any color in particular, but I prefer black and white." It's her sense of experimentation and a taste for adventure that lends itself well to devising a whole new look for Penny.

PENNY McGARRY

HAIR ANALYSIS
Texture: Straight and thick
Condition: Healthy
Percentage of Silver: Twenty-five

FACE ANALYSIS
Skin Condition: Normal
Wrinkles: Almost none
Sun Damage: Limited to a few freckles

COLOR PALETTE: Cool

BEAUTY BONUSES: Excellent skin; large pretty eyes

AREAS TO TROUBLESHOOT: Long face, no visible cheekbones

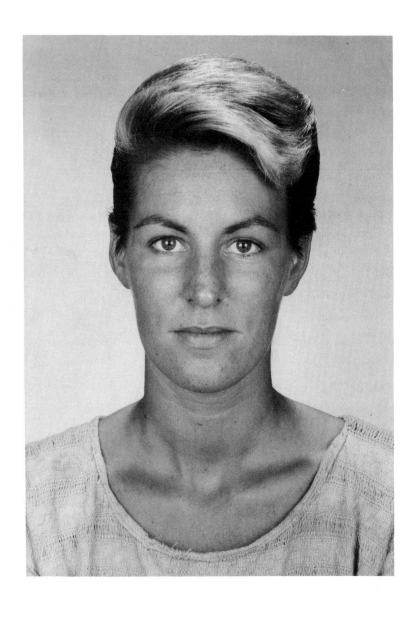

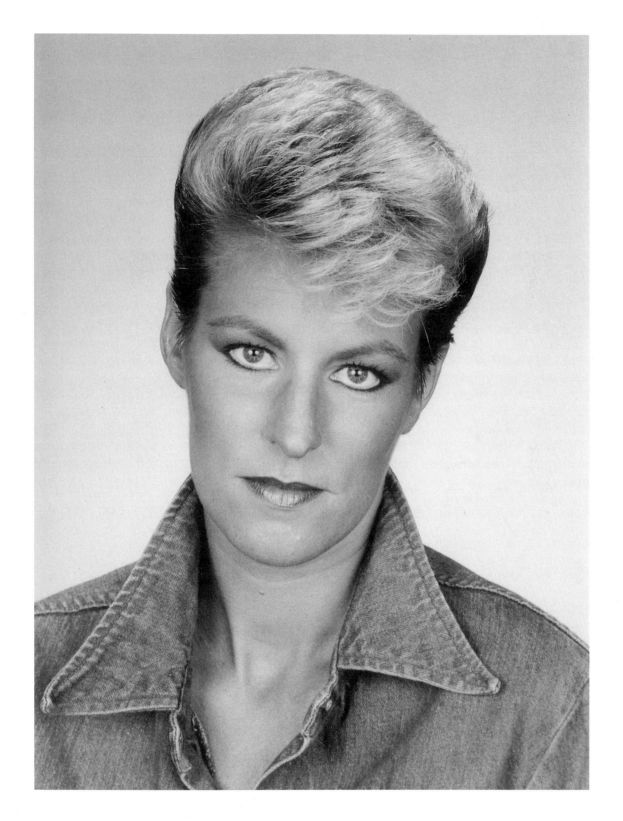

PENNY McGARRY'S MAKEOVER

Penny's silver grew in in streaks on top and at the sides. To create a dramatic effect, she covered the sides with ash-brown semipermanent color and left the top light. I decided to add a few more silvery highlights on top to enhance the contrast even further. Penny is young enough to be able to play a little with her silver.

The severe cut suited her well, but it had even more versatility than she realized. After washing it, I combed an egg-sized portion of styling mousse through her hair and blow dried it into this sleek, modern pompadour.

You saw another look with exactly this cut on page 205. To get this effect, I partially rough blow-dried her hair. Then I styled it into a free, full style for short hair. To do this, I needed a styling glaze (in this case, Vidal Sassoon's Body Glaze). I applied it to her semidamp hair at the roots and distributed it throughout by twisting strands of hair up and back. I pulled a few strands down to play up her eyes—the effect was slick and sassy!

Penny didn't need any concealer—rose-beige foundation was enough to even out her lightly freckled complexion.

Her face is oblong and lacking in definition, so we "invented" cheekbones for her. Two tones of blush did the trick: a soft burgundy *under* the bone and swept up to her temples, and a lighter pink *on* the bone.

You saw us make her eyes earlier in the book. It's our classic daytime look in cool shades of shell-pink highlighter, smoky-lavender contour, and wine accent colors, with charcoal liner and mascara.

Penny's upper lip is a little thin, so we lined it just outside her natural line with a blue-red pencil, then lined the lower lip on its natural line. We colored with raspberry lipstick applied with a slant-tipped lip brush.

In an all-American, washed-out-denim jacket, Penny looks fresh and youthful.

Index